CARNIVORE DIET

A Guide to Eat Meat, Get Lean, and Stay Healthy an Alternative for Paleo and Keto Diet

JACOB GREENE

Table of Contents

INTRODUCTION

I want to thank you for choosing this book, '*Carnivore Diet - A Guide to Eat Meat, Get Lean, and Stay Healthy.*'

If you are someone who loves a juicy steak or just about any type of meat, this is the right book for you. Here, we are going to delve deep into a diet that will challenge what you know about nutrition and health and will let you explore some new possibilities. This diet, as the title suggests, is the carnivore diet. A lot of you may or may not be familiar with what this diet is all about, but it will all be explained in the book nonetheless.

The main emphasis of the carnivore diet is to eat only meat from any source and stop eating food from plant sources. This diet has gained a lot of popularity lately, and the strong motivation behind this diet is usually weight loss. Many people follow this diet to address a certain type of autoimmune system, where meat diets are beneficial.

A lot of people try the Carnivore diet after they have tried the Paleo and the Ketogenic diet. As you might know, the Paleo diet is a caveman diet that focuses on eating fresh food like our ancestors in the caveman era ate. It eliminates all processed food, grains, dairy, sugars, etc., which were not available at the time. The Ketogenic diet, on the other hand, is focused on a major reduction of carbohydrates from the diet with a high intake of fat and moderate intake of protein. The diet is best for people who want a higher protein intake and want to limit their fat or carb intake.

As you read the book, you will understand what the carnivore diet entails exactly. The meat only diet is quite self-explanatory, but there are a few gray areas that you can work with to create a suitable healthy diet for yourself. This diet has been tried by a lot of people and if followed appropriately, can benefit you in losing weight and getting healthier. If you are a meat lover, this diet is like a dream come true for you.

CHAPTER ONE -

WHAT IS THE CARNIVORE DIET?

Let's imagine your meals for a particular day this week, a plate of bacon for breakfast, a sizzling steak for lunch and a juicy beef burger patty for dinner. Does this sound appealing to you? Well, this is what the carnivore diet usually looks like, and you can eat these meals guilt free when you follow it. The only quirk is that there won't be any side veggies or burger buns or even any type of processed cheese on your burger. If you can live without these extra ingredients, the carnivore diet will work well for you.

The carnivore diet is also known as a zero-carb diet, carnivorous diet or the all meat diet and has one simple principle; you can only eat meat. Essentially, you are supposed to eat almost nothing other than meat for every single meal every day as long as you are following the diet. This diet will not dictate your portions, calories, food timings or macro percentage. You are allowed to eat whenever you are hungry and as much as you need to feel full. There are certain gray areas that a follower of the diet can customize according to their preference.

For instance, some people add ingredients like cream or cheese to their diet while others place a complete restriction on consuming anything other than meat. According to the guidelines of the diet, you may eat animal sourced food that includes meat, eggs or dairy. You can consume as much protein and fat as you must from these foods, but carbohydrates should be excluded from the diet.

The carnivore diet is especially beneficial because of the carbohydrate-eliminating factor. There are certain places around the world where people actually survive on zero carbohydrates and instead eat according to the carnivore diet. It is not because they are following a fad diet but is a practice they have followed for as far back as they can remember. It might sound extreme to you when you think of surviving only on meat, fish, etc. with absolutely no grains or such carbohydrates. This is mostly because your usual diet includes grains as a staple and you've been told that they are healthy for your heart. However, research shows that the introduction of refined carbohydrates is what caused a huge increase in the rates of diabetes, hypertension, tooth cavities and atherosclerosis in people. This is why a lot of people these days try eliminating carbs from their diet.

Another major factor is that excess carb consumption is a major cause of weight gain. To be honest, eliminating carbs will work for some people while for some it may not. You can adjust your diet accordingly to suit your body's needs. Reducing carbs in your diet will aid you in weight loss and other health issues, but it is a macro that needs limiting and doesn't always need complete elimination.

Many studies have been conducted to see the effects of a low carbohydrate diet on people. These show that reducing carbs helps to enhance mental performance, increase physical endurance, support digestion and also reduce inflammation in the body. A low carb diet is also really good for cardiovascular health. Another benefit is that it boosts energy while unhealthy food cravings are reduced. All these factors together show that the no-carb carnivore diet can improve health and reduce weight too. This diet is just one of the more hardcore versions of low-carb or high-fat diets like Paleo and Keto diets. In this carnivore version, instead of just reducing carbs, there is a complete elimination of this macro from the diet.

The carnivore diet has cultural precedence as we mentioned earlier. For instance, in Eskimo groups, their diet mostly consisted of a fish, walrus or whales as a high-fat animal sourced diet. Even in the Masai region of Africa, the diet consists majorly of meat with milk. These people have shown to have very low levels of bad cholesterol and low rates of cardiovascular diseases as well.

If you want real researched proof about the effects of the carnivore diet, there are unfortunately not enough long-term formal studies completed yet; however, there are many thriving communities online that you can go through to find out more about the real-life effects of this diet.

A lot of the people who have followed the carnivore diet leave testimonials or comments on how it worked out for them. You can always use these to judge if the diet suits your needs or not; however, ultimately, the best way to know for certain is to follow the diet yourself and experience it. The diet can be quite tempting if you are not a fan of salad greens but love your portion of meat.

CHAPTER TWO -

BACKGROUND HISTORY OF THE CARNIVORE DIET

According to the people who advocate the benefits of the carnivore diet, there is a simple reason behind its effectiveness. The reason that our ancestors preferred to eat most of the time because gathering fruit and vegetables took up a lot of energy. Hunting and eating meat were much more energy efficient. Due to this carnivorous diet followed by our ancestors, our bodies evolved in a way that they run at the most optimal level when our diet is meat-centric. This is one of the main theories behind which the carnivore diet is supported.

In recorded history, there are many examples of people from a variety of ethnic, cultural or even geographical backgrounds that survived on a meat-centric diet and remained quite healthy throughout their lifetime. On the other hand, no civilization has been noted to follow a purely vegan diet through generations. There has to be a reason behind which most people through the ages preferred meat as the main component in their diets.

These days, there are a lot of stigmas against meat. A lot of people seem to be advocating a vegetarian or vegan or even fruitarian diet that is free of all meat or animal-sourced food. We are told that meat is the reason behind artery clogging, weight gain, high levels of cholesterol, constipation, etc. Thus, you should give up meat and follow a solely plant-based diet; however, no civilization has people who have survived healthily on a vegan diet from childhood until old age.

If you consider it anthropologically, the real-world examples of various cultures following a particular diet is much more valid than any scientific studies that are conducted to understand something. The fact that people thrived on the carnivore diet through the ages is a much more valid testimony that the information gathered by a scientific study conducted on a few people over a few weeks. The former is a more realistic way of looking at the diet than the latter, which will involve a group of people eating more meat than usual for some time while a study is being conducted.

There have been studies conducted to specifically show that a diet with fewer animal products is healthier than one with more of it; however, these studies have mostly failed to prove it since a non-vegetarian culture is not less healthy in any way compared to a vegetarian culture. Animal foods are quite essential for the health of a human being. If you take a look at different groups all around the world and study their history as well, you will see that every healthy community survives on at least a few animal foods if not a lot. There is no healthy group of people with complete independence from animal-sourced foods.

Like we mentioned before two specific groups in the world are used as a prime example of a healthy carnivorous community. The first group is the Eskimos who eat meat and fat almost exclusively. People who lived in the Arctic regions saw a change in their diet only around the latter part of the 1800s when trade routes were being built extensively. This provided them access to sugar, flour and other European foods that were then introduced into their original diet; however, before this change in their diet, they were healthier on the diet that primarily consisted of animal protein with fat. The second group is the Masai people of Africa who eat very little plant foods and survive mostly on meat, milk and even blood of animals. The herdsmen from these regions in Africa ate more meat when they were age 14-30 since these were their warrior years. More meat was considered crucial to stronger bodies and thus would be beneficial for a warrior. It is to be noted though that the old cultures that adopted this kind of meat-centric diet did so to adapt to certain extreme environmental factors. Most of the groups around the world who followed a carnivorous diet resided in desert, arctic or sub-arctic regions. The food is scarce in such areas, and the availability of food is unpredictable as well.

Many other communities survive on a meat-based diet as well; for instance - the Inuit of the Canadian Arctic region. Their diet consists mostly of fish, walrus, whale and seal meat. In the Russian Arctic, the Chukotka people live on a diet of marine creatures, caribou meat, and fish. In East Africa, the Samburu, as well as the Rendille people, have survived for years on a meat and milk diet. In Mongolia, the Steppe nomads usually eat dairy products and meat daily. In South Dakota, the Sioux are known to have buffalo meat as the staple in their diet. Beef is the main part of meals for the Brazilian Gauchos.

As you can see, a carnivorous diet has been followed all over the world for a very long time, and these people have enjoyed healthy lives through generations despite the stigma against meat. The dogma that exists about saturated fat and cholesterol from meat in the American diet is completely discredited. The groups of people in the Arctic and African tribes that eat meat filled diet do not have any recorded instances of heart diseases or such ailments in the past and these increased only when modern foods were introduced in their diets.

If you take time to look at the diet of the ethnic groups that exist in the Arctic region, you will see that they consume barely any amount of fruit or vegetables all year around. Doesn't that make you wonder how they survive or manage to live healthy lives? You probably doubt that they received sufficient amounts of the essential vitamins and minerals in their diet then; however, they have lived like this for a very long time and thrived on this diet as they still do today.

One of the prominent studies that support the carnivore diet is one conducted by a dentist from Cleveland by the name of Weston A. Price. He started an investigation that he carried out on the subject for nearly a decade. From his profession, he observed how most people suffered from dental issues and other metabolic conditions. He noticed all the health issues and even the facial deformities that kept increasing in the number of patients he saw. He was curious about the cause of these problems because he believed that God was not the one who would allow this kind of suffering among his people. This curiosity and interest prompted him to research the root cause of all these diseases. At that point 60 years ago, there was no one else who had given this much thought. He was the only one who wanted to study various civilizations around the world and learn the cause of the health issues he came across in different people. He went from the Swiss region to Africa, Australia and many more places around the world.

Everything he observed and studied, he noted down in his published book called "Nutrition and Physical Degeneration." This book was quite eye opening to the people who read it. Price's focus was on the food habits of ethnic groups from different parts across the globe, which was relatively untouched by the modern diet. He saw that these people displayed very good physical health and there was barely any incidence of the modern-day diseases that are common in the outside regions. He was surprised by this and was curious about how they could be in such good health without any aid from modern medicine. The key to all his questions lies in the eating habits of these isolated ethnic groups. His observation was that they all had a diet that barely had any plant produce and was mostly based on animal-sourced products. His study was just another proof of the fact that meat is a very healthy component of the human diet and should not be eliminated. A meat-centric diet has sufficient amounts of the required nutrients and minerals that are required for optimal physical health.

Another study to be noted is one that was conducted nearly 40 years ago in Point Hope, Alaska. The place is very isolated, and this was why they were still on a very meat focused diet. The study was published in the year 1972 and gave various observations based on their diet and health. It said that the people of Point Hope were one of the very few remaining cultures that survived on the Eskimo diet. Their daily calorie intake was averaged at 3000 kcal per person, and half of this was from fat while about 35% was from protein. Only a maximum of 20% of their calories was derived from carbohydrates that were in the form of animal starch. Their diet scarcely had any grain and the only time sucrose was ingested when a little was added to tea or coffee. The research showed that the residents of Point Hope had nearly ten times lower incidence of heart disease compared to the rest of the general population in the United States of America. You can see from this that meat does not have a negative impact on your cardiovascular health as you are told these days. Yet Vilhjalmur Stefansson conducted another meat-based diet research on the Inuit people between the years 1906 and 1919. He described this research in his book called "The Fat of the Land."

According to this study, the Inuit eat a completely meat-based diet all year round. Under some rare circumstances, they might eat some plant foods like berries, which were preserved for eating in the winter. If no meat was available, they sometimes ate vegetables as a last resort. The anthropologist himself tried the diet for a while but could not stick to it; however, in his study, he told of how the Inuit people of both genders and all ages were leading healthy thriving lives while surviving on 100% meat. The study also said that these people were free from scurvy and other meat-related diseases that the modern civilization fears. They don't even consume any salt with their meat yet have no issues related to sodium or electrolyte levels in their body. The study too demonstrated how traditional groups like these thrived on the carnivore diet and were in robust health.

As you keep reading this book, you will see how the carnivore diet works and why it is beneficial for you even in this day and age.

CHAPTER THREE -

BENEFITS OF THE CARNIVORE DIET

If you need to be convinced further about trying the carnivore diet, this section of the book will help you out. There are various benefits that you will experience when you follow this meat-based diet appropriately.

Weight loss - A lot of people doubt it when they hear that a completely meat-based diet will help them lose weight or even benefit their health; however, as you learn more about it, you will understand exactly why it is true. Let me tell you that this diet requires you to abstain from consuming carbohydrates. When your carbohydrate consumption is low, so are your blood sugar levels, and thus this prevents insulin spikes. This, in turn, will prevent calories from being deposited in your body in the form of fats which then leads to weight gain or even obesity. Reducing carbs on a diet also helps you in avoiding excessive calorie consumption and reduces unhealthy eating as well. Your body only needs as many calories as it requires for energy during your daily activities.

If you don't burn much but consume more calories, this will just get stored in the body. This is why the carbohydrate deficiency in the Carnivore diet will help you in losing weight. Instead, it helps to increase the amount of proteins and fats you consume, and this will help to satisfy your appetite for longer. Unhealthy cravings or hunger pangs will also reduce.

A lot of people gain weight without realizing it because they eat absent-mindedly.

The carnivore diet helps to reduce this as well because you will not feel hungry all the time and thus eat more mind-fully when you are hungry. If you think about it, the foods that we eat while watching TV, reading a book, etc. are usually junk foods that we just keep shoving int our mouths. When your diet is restricted to meat, you are hardly likely to keep snacking on a steak or any other type of meat.

In time, as you follow the diet, it will help you differentiate between actual hunger and psychological hunger. On this diet, you can't reach out for a bag of chips at any time you want, so even without any calorie counting, your calorie intake is reduced. Reducing the carbohydrate intake will also push your body into ketosis like in the Ketogenic diet. Your body will then burn fat for energy and help you lose weight even more. If you want a summary of how you lose weight on this diet, consider the following. It makes you eat more protein and drink more water. It limits the types of foods you can eat and also reduces oil, sugar or flour. You will instead be eating food that is higher volume, and this will lead to chew better and aid in digestion. Thus, the diet will aid in weight loss.

Cardiovascular health

 A few decades ago, meat and even eggs started being blamed for the increasing incidence of heart diseases; however, we know it is not as simple as that. When it comes to meat, processed meat is usually linked to heart diseases and not red meat. It is not just the cholesterol in foods that you should pay attention to but also the amount of saturated fat in it. Eating too much-processed foods or carbohydrates will cause an increase in the level of LDL in your body. LDL is the bad cholesterol that needs to be reduced in your body while HDL is the good cholesterol that your heart will benefit from. When the LDL levels increase, it affects your cardiovascular health negatively; however, on the Carnivore diet, you will increase the HDL levels and thus improve the condition of your heart.

Reduction of inflammation

Your liver will produce something called C-reactive proteins or CRP in case of inflammation in your body. The level of this CRP indicates the amount of inflammation in your body. It is a myth that animal-sourced foods cause inflammation. Reducing the intake of plant-sourced foods will reduce the amount of inflammation that is indicated by high CRP levels. You should take note of any particular plant foods that cause inflammation in your body and take care to cut those out from your diet. Thus, a meat-based diet will help to reduce inflammation, and this will aid in reducing pain in the joints or from arthritis.

Increases testosterone levels

Consuming more fat in your diet will automatically help to boost the amount of testosterone in your body. Studies proved this by comparing men who had a high-fat diet with men who had a low-fat diet. Thus, the carnivore diet is beneficial for men to increase healthy testosterone levels as well.

Improves digestion

The digestive system is a major cause for concern if your diet is unhealthy. A lot of people advocate that high amounts of fiber in the diet are essential for digestive health; however, this is not necessarily true. A study showed that reducing fiber could benefit your digestive system. The carnivore diet can thus help to treat constipation, improving bowel movements and reducing bloating or gas as well.

Improves focus and clarity

If you are familiar with the Ketogenic diet, you will know that it aids in improving the functioning of the brain and increases focus or mental clarity. Similarly, the carnivore diet does the same as well and pushes your body into ketosis. A lot of people notice an energy drop in the afternoon on this usual modern-day diet; however, this can be prevented as the carnivore diet helps stabilize energy levels and keeps you functioning optimally throughout the day. Since the fats in your body are the main source of energy, you don't need to keep eating to replenish your energy source.

Better oral health

Sugar has a very unhealthy impact on your oral health. It is one of the main causes of cavities and also causes an imbalance in pH levels in the mouth. The carnivore diet cuts out sugar from your diet, and this helps to restore a healthy pH level. It will also prevent bacteria from breeding in your mouth and causing any infection or decay in your teeth. A lot of people also suffer from gum disease and the carnivore diet helps to manage it and treat it over time.

Improved eyesight

You might question this but trust us when we say that sugar has a very bad impact on your eyesight as well. When you eliminate sugar from your diet, the levels in your body reduce as well. This then reduces the risk of cataracts and helps to keep your eyes healthy.

Simplifies your diet

Unlike some other complicated fad diets, the carnivore diet is very easy to implement. There are no fancy ingredients or foods you need to source. The only food you need is meat or animal-sourced food. You don't have to bother about macros, food diaries, calorie counting, etc. There is no stress about planning or shopping for a carnivore diet.

As you can see, there are numerous positive changes that the carnivore diet will bring in your body and life in general. We think you should try the diet and see for yourself if these work for you like they have for many others.

CHAPTER FOUR -

THE EFFECTS OF THE CARNIVORE DIET ON DIGESTION

Your digestive system plays a major role in your body. Your diet has a major impact on your digestion in turn. This is why it is important to pay due heed to the effects of the various foods you eat on your digestion. Every system in your body is interlinked, and a problem with one will also cause health issues in other regards. This section will help you understand the effect of the carnivore diet on the digestive system.

Every healthy gut has a couple of kilograms of microbes in it. These include nearly a thousand different species of bacteria, and the health of these microbes will affect your digestive health. Bacteria are not always bad. The ones that are naturally in your stomach aid in the digestive process and are essential for good gut health. They help your body to absorb nutrients from the food that is being digested. The small intestine and stomach cannot ingest every type of food. At this point, the microbes come in and do it for them. This is why it is important to support good microbe health in your gut. The foods you eat will determine this. Some foods will aid in this and others will cause a negative reaction.

Processed food and sugar is not good for your digestive system. This is why the carnivore diet requires you to eliminate any such foods and focus on healthy fat and meat-based food. Sugars and processed food will cause undesirable bacteria to grow in your gut. This will cause an imbalance in a healthy microbiome system in your gut. Your digestive system is affected, and food is not digested optimally. The good bacteria in your gut are harmed by all the sugars, artificial sweeteners and ingredients in processed food. This is why they need to be eliminated if you want the probiotic bacteria to thrive in your digestive system while eliminating harmful bacteria.

A leaky gut can be another problem in an unhealthy digestive system. The carnivore diet also aids in preventing this and restoring health. In the food you eat, not every substance is desirable for your body. The good bacteria and a healthy gut make sure that these stay within the gastrointestinal tract since they act as a barrier. When your gut lining is not in a healthy condition, the barrier is also not effective. This means that the harmful substances can escape from the gastrointestinal tract and get into the bloodstream. This can be a very dangerous situation for your body. It is not just harmful bacteria that get into your bloodstream but food particles and toxins as well. This is why it is important to pay attention to gut health so that a healthy barrier is maintained.

A leaky gut will show adverse effects on various aspects of your body. This includes your skin, hormones as well as your brain. You might wonder how the carnivore diet aids in preventing this. The restriction of foods therefore plays an important role. Grains, as well as legumes, can cause weakening of the barrier. The gluten in these foods can be a major cause of autoimmune disorders. There is a protein molecule called Zonulin that is activated by gluten from grains. This protein molecule breaks the bonds between the cells within the intestinal walls and gut lining. The lectins and phytic acids in these foods also weaken the barrier and are thus bad for gut health. These foods can also end up being a cause of leaky gut syndrome that is a very harmful digestive condition that you need to prevent. The carnivore diet does not include any of these grains or legumes, so it does not harm the gut lining. The dietary fats will instead help to release proteins that will strengthen the gut by reducing inflammation.

The modern western diet is sadly lacking in terms of healthy dietary fats. People have reduced their fat intake as much as possible since they believe it is the culprit behind weight gain and other health issues. The truth is that carbohydrates are the cause and fats are healthy. These carbs should be eliminated instead, and the carnivore diet helps to do this. Instead, you are encouraged to eat food that has a lot of dietary fat like meat and other dairy products. Eating grass-fed meat along with seafood will give you a regular healthy supply of omega 3 fatty acids. These are healthy and increase the diversity of the bacteria that are essential for proper digestion. This microbiome unit in the stomach is quite like a small ecosystem by itself and diversity is always a good way to evolve. The more your diet comprises of healthy fats, the more diverse it will be, and thus it is better for your health.

Nearly all the health problems suffered by these few generations have been caused by the unhealthy modern diet and lifestyle. The way we eat, how we live all affects us negatively and thus causes illness. The food in the modern diet is full of GMOs, pesticides, chemicals, additives, etc. and these damages your gut as a whole. When you switch to the basic way of eating followed by our ancestors, you will improve the health of the digestive system. The more processed food you eat, the worse it gets. The carnivore diet will help to prevent such unhealthy conditions.

If you are worried about the lack of fiber in the diet, you should not be. Most of us have been told that fiber is essential for a healthy digestive system and regular bowel movements. The carnivore diet lacks this factor; however, fiber is not as important as it is made out to be. Instead of fiber, the healthy fat in your food will help in bowel regulation. These dietary fats ease the process of waste elimination from the body. You might notice that it is less frequent than usual, but this is normal. The carnivore diet itself is the reason behind it. Your body just does not need to get rid of as much waste as it does in the usual diet. It is true that fiber is important for certain people due to their particular genetic makeup, but it is not necessary for everyone to consume a high fiber diet.

You must know that every system in the body is interlinked in some way or the other, so the digestive system is also linked to the brain. Your gut works as a new brain in your body. This is why people say, "Go with your gut" when you have to make some decisions. There is a lot of research that says that the gut and mind are quite connected. Your gut is strongly linked to your emotions even if you might not have thought of it before. Have you noticed how your stomach seems to ache when you are scared or nervous or how there is a sensation like butterflies moving at times? This is why there are so many sayings related to the gut. There is scientific reasoning behind this too. The enteric nervous system or ENS is present in the gut. This ENS has control over secretions and blood flow within the gastrointestinal tract. Due to this system, you can feel what is happening in your gut. This is why the gut has a lot of control over digestion in your body.

When you experience stress, even this is connected to the functioning of your gut. Are you familiar with the fight or flight instinct? This is an instinct in humans that help them to protect themselves. This instinct is responsible for the regulation of cortisol level in your body. The body functions normally when there is no stress. But when you are experiencing stress, the body also experiences this fight or flight emotion.

The human body seems incapable of differentiating between physical and psychological stress. If you are someone who deals with chronic stress or anxiety, you are at high risk of chronic inflammation. The same way that your body reacts if there is an infection, it will react in case of stress. It is important to try and alleviate such stress from your daily life if you want to prevent the damage from inflammation on your system. Pay heed to the connection between your mind and gut. The body has a way of letting you know when it is in distress so that you can make an effort to take care of it. If you eat a healthy diet like the carnivore diet, it will improve your gut health and also ensure good mental health. The leaky gut syndrome we mentioned earlier could even cause mental fog so beware of these symptoms. Improving gut health will restore mental clarity.

CHAPTER FIVE -

THE EFFECT OF THE CARNIVORE DIET ON CHOLESTEROL

A common misconception is that eating meat, butter or even eggs is one of the main causes of high levels of bad cholesterol. You will hear a lot of so-called weight gurus telling you to stop eating any of these if you want to lose weight or improve your health. You probably doubt the validity of us saying that a diet rich in these foods won't affect your health in any way and especially in terms of alcohol. It might make you feel like we are saying that eating a lot of junk food won't make you fat. But on an honest note, the two are in no way similar.

Cholesterol itself has many misconceptions associated with it. In this section, we will try and explain more about how your diet will affect your cholesterol levels and if you should be worried or not. But before you do this, you have to keep an open mind and let go of the misconceptions you already have. Only then will you understand how it works and why the carnivore diet is healthy for you.

Most of what we know about cholesterol is not true and is just based on unreasonable statements made by certain people who themselves don't understand any better. Cholesterol is a wax-like substance that is produced by humans and animals. No other living form produces cholesterol; so, all plant sources are free of it. A lot of research has shown that people with clogged arteries are more likely to suffer from cardiovascular health issues. There is a direct link between the arteries and heart, and it affects your health.

The more clogged your arteries are, the higher your chances of suffering from a stroke or cardiac arrest. From this research, they concluded cholesterol was to blame for heart issues since it was what clogged the arteries. This is why people were told that if they ate foods rich in cholesterol, it would increase levels in their body and thus cause heart ailments. Naturally, people started demonizing red meat, butter, eggs and such cholesterol rich food.

However, do high cholesterol foods affect the levels in your body? The answer is no because your body already knows how to control levels of cholesterol. Since the human body itself produces cholesterol, it has its mechanism to maintain healthy levels in the body. It works like a feedback mechanism where the body stops producing cholesterol when it notices there are high levels of it already. Similarly, if the level of cholesterol decreases, the body produces more of it.

What you need to understand is that cholesterol is not all bad. It has its classification of good cholesterol and bad cholesterol. This is what you need to pay attention to. Cholesterol exists as a fat molecule that isn't soluble like salt or sugar. This is why it needs a medium to travel through the body since it will not dissolve in the blood itself. This medium used by cholesterol molecules is lipoproteins. They are a mixed molecule group, which contains both protein and fat. The main function of lipoproteins is cholesterol transport to organs or cells when required. Among lipoproteins, there is a classification of two types that are responsible for this cholesterol transport. One is high-density lipoprotein or

HDL, and the other is low-density lipoprotein or LDL. Although the HDL and LDL can't technically be called cholesterol, they are known as good and bad cholesterol.

The function of HDL molecules is to transport cholesterol from different parts of your body to your liver. In the liver, it is either removed or reused for the body. The LDL molecules transport cholesterol from the liver to the rest of the body. If the level of HDL or good cholesterol is high in your body, you risk of cardiovascular diseases is lower. To increase the level of HDL, your diet should be rich in natural dietary fibers. This is why a low carbohydrate diet has a positive effect by increasing HDL levels.

On the other hand, the LDL level should not be high, and this is why it is called bad cholesterol; however, it is just a low-density lipoprotein and not actual cholesterol. The LDL itself is responsible for transporting cholesterol, and when the level of this is high, more cholesterol is taken to the liver. Increased LDL levels are responsible for the higher risk of heart ailments. The smaller LDL particles further contribute to this negative impact. When you consume a low carb diet, it helps to turn these into larger molecules and also cause a reduction of LDL in the blood. By now you can understand that a dietary fat-rich diet will not cause issues in cholesterol. This kind of diet facilitates a more balanced cholesterol level in the body.

Just like cholesterol, people are also wary of triglyceride levels. But most of the fears related to triglycerides are quite baseless. Triglycerides are a type of fat that is most commonly found in food. They help to provide fuel for the body. The only difference is that they are used as fuel storage for the future and not for immediate use by the body. When your body is breaking down sugars to use for energy, some of it is stored in cells as triglycerides. The more the body deals with carbohydrates, the more insulin it produces. Too much of insulin will cause problems with blood sugar in the body, and this will then increase the stored triglyceride levels. So, it is not about the fats that you need to worry again. Eating a diet low in carbs will help to prevent any such problems. This is why the carnivore diet eliminates carbs and helps to maintain good health.

Don't let myths and misconceptions about cholesterol and triglycerides mislead you. It is important to learn the scientific reasoning behind something before believing what is told in general. A half-truth is equal to a lie and can be harmful. When you learn more about something, it helps you understand it better. This is why we are making an effort to explain the details of the carnivore diet and its effect on the body to you. This book is not just some blank guide that tells you to do this and that while making false claims. We are here to help you understand how things work in your body and why we recommend this particular diet to help you lose unwanted weight, get lean and stay healthy for a long time.

CHAPTER SIX -

HOW TO START THE CARNIVORE DIET?

If you want to try the carnivore diet for yourself, you have to understand that you won't get instant results. Any healthy diet requires at least a few weeks to kick in and show results. To begin the carnivore diet, you can start with a one-month target. If you see it working and don't notice any bad side effects, you can continue from there on. Take notes on how you feel throughout that month in terms of things like energy, hunger cravings, etc. and also mark your weight down every week. You can use this time to be subjective about the diet and see how it works for you. A health diary is a great way to mark down progress and stay motivated. In this section, we will try to help you in the process of beginning the carnivore diet.

Stages of the Carnivore Diet

The carnivore diet can be divided into three stages, and this section will help you learn about them. When you start the carnivore diet, you can opt to go one stage at a time or just begin from the second stage if it suits you better. We will help you understand what every stage involves and more.

<u>Stage One</u>

At this stage, you can eat every kind of meat or seafood that you want. There is no restriction on tea or coffee. You are allowed to eat cheese, butter, eggs, and even heavy cream. This is the stage that allows your body to get adapted to the carnivore diet, and you are also allowed to add some supplements to aid you in the transition. Electrolytes are also recommended to counter the diuretic effect on the body caused by the carnivore diet; however, even if you use salt, it should be kosher. This kosher salt rule applies for any stage during the diet.

Stage Two

Whatever you do in stage one is allowed on stage two with two exceptions. You have to exclude all processed meats at this point in the diet. This includes all the ham, cold cut salami, sausages, etc. You also have to stop drinking coffee and tea since there was enough time in the adaptation period to get rid of the habit; however, this second aspect is not as important as giving up processed meat which is not healthy for you.

Stage Three

At this point in the diet, it is a little harder for you, but it needs to be worked through if you want the carnivore diet to work optimally for you. Eliminate all foods and beverages in your diet except beef and water. A lot of research has shown that beef is the healthiest option while following this diet. Since we also eliminated processed meat, you need to find a place that will supply you with organic grass-fed meat. Give up any other meat or seafood other than beef at this stage; however, don't stress about the grass-fed source if it is too expensive. Just try to stick to eating only beef with water. There are different cuts of beef that you can keep switching up so that you don't get bored with the diet.

Follow these three stages in the first 30 days of beginning the carnivore diet. Don't try tinkering with the diet at this point so that you adapt well and it works optimally for you. After the 30 days, you are allowed to personalize it to suit your lifestyle and needs. Experiment with the foods that are allowed and see what works best for you. You will notice that even within the diet, some types of food will help to lose weight while others might make you gain a little. So limit your intake accordingly when you are trying to maintain a healthier body.

When you start personalizing after stage three, do it step by step. Start by adding regular beef to your grass-fed beef diet. Then start adding other animal meat or seafood as well; however, go with the addition of one meat at a time. After this you can start introducing eggs to your diet, followed by the other permitted dairy products. Test what works for you and what doesn't. In the end, you can also start drinking a little tea or coffee if you managed to cut the habit by stage two.

When you are introducing a single food at a time, it allows you time to notice how your body reacts to that particular food. If you see any unfavorable effect, try to limit or restrict consumption of it. This is why a lot of people omit pork when they see that it causes a bit of weight gain. You can also omit a food if there are any other ill effects like food allergies. In the case of some dairy products, you may notice bloating. In this case, you should eliminate the food that induces bloating in your body; however, when it comes to eggs, we recommend including it in your diet. Other than all this, go ahead and personalize your diet plan according to your goals. Be patient and go through all the stages one at a time.

On a more general note, other than following stages mentioned above, follow the points given below as a guide.

What to Eat

First off, you need to find out everything that you are allowed to eat on this diet. Anything not on the Carnivore diet list should not be consumed at least for the one month that you have set the target for. As you already know by now, primarily you are only allowed to eat animal meat. It is a 100% meat meal diet. There is no space for any plant-based foods or even plant sources of protein like soy protein. As you will learn later in the book, certain dairy products are allowed on an occasional basis, but even this can be eliminated if you choose.

Get rid of all the processed food from your kitchen or pantry before you stock up on your meat-centric food list. There should be no plant-sourced foods either, so you can give away your food to your friend or even to the homeless shelter nearby. Remember that there should be no sugar, sauces and other condiments in your diet either. Unless someone else in your house is going to consume all this, get it out of your sight. This will prevent you from relapsing into your old habits.

How much to Eat

After you are certain of the foods that are permitted on the Carnivore diet, you can stock up on them and start. At this point, you might be worried about how much you are allowed to eat or aren't. Well, the great thing about this diet is that there are no restrictions on the quantity of food. Of course, you should not overeat, but you can eat until you feel satiated. Don't try to starve yourself just because you think that it will help you lose weight. Eat when you are hungry because it is the body's way of telling you it needs more energy and nourishment. You will learn to differentiate real hunger from psychological hunger as you start the meat diet.

During this first month, you will see changes in the pattern of your appetite. Your cravings and untimely hunger will reduce and be replaced with a more appropriate dietary habit. This will also help you in the process of eating less and burning fat. You can judge the amount of food you need in a day by the amount of activity you do. If you have a more sedentary life, eat enough meat to keep you going through the day but avoid eating too much.

If you are a very active person or take part in regular sports, you might even need the double amount of food compared to the average person. Accordingly, you can decide for yourself how much food you need. On some days you can eat lesser than another day when you eat more because you were very active all day. You have to remember and eat only when you are hungry and eat until you feel satisfied. Don't try to eat less and stay hungry. Instead, eat your fill during a meal and avoid eating in between. Don't try to stuff yourself with too much either, learn to listen to your body. It will help you understand when you need food and when you don't. Ideally, you can eat 2-4 lbs of meat in a day.

When to Eat

The next thing to consider is what time or when you should eat. Ideally, three main meals in the day are more than enough. You should also try to set a schedule so that you eat at the same time every day, as this will benefit your health further. Any individual's timing will depend on their daily schedule. Try to ensure that you eat a healthy protein-based breakfast in the morning to stabilize your energy levels throughout the day. No matter how busy you are at work, set aside time to eat your lunch. Carry your own from home so that you can avoid breaking the restrictions of your diet. Also, practice mindful eating and don't try to multitask and work while you eat lunch. Once you are home, you can have dinner a few hours before you go to bed. If you feel hungry in between any meal, try drinking water and if you are still hungry eat a little food. But remember to stick to the diet approved foods at all times.

What to drink

Preferably, you should only drink water when you are on the carnivore diet. At least for this first month of trial, avoid drinking any other liquid. Don't buy any packaged drinks that say low fat, no sugar or health drink either. Only drink water, this can be tap water, spring water, mineral water or even filtered water but nothing with added flavoring or sugars. If you can't give up on your regular dose of coffee or tea, make sure you don't add any sugar or artificial sweeteners to it. You will have to give these up for the second and third stage of the diet but many continue afterwards. Any sodas, juices, protein shakes, etc. are out of limits in this diet. Water is always the best way to stay hydrated n matter what diet you are on. It aids in losing weight faster and will prevent bloating from water retention.

How to Cook

Usually, there is no strict guideline about the way you cook. If you like your steak rare, eat it that way, but if you prefer it well done, this works too. No matter what meat or fish you are cooking, just make sure it is done in a way that the food is safe to eat. Certain types of meat will make you ill if left uncooked and consumed. On the other hand, there are a few types that can be consumed raw as well. For instance, you can eat raw sushi salmon or fresh oysters if you like. Also, since you are eating meat most of the time, invest in some good meat cutting knives and a board that is meant for this purpose. Vegetable knives are quite difficult to use when you want to slice certain types of tough cuts.

Common Mistakes You should avoid

A lot of people who want to lose weight often eat too little even when the diet does not restrict food quantity. Starving yourself will not make you healthily lose weight and will instead cause illness. Eat enough to satiate your hunger, and over time you will find that the diet itself helps to normalize your appetite. You also have to remember and stay hydrated throughout the day. This is to prevent dehydration and aid in healthy bodily functions. Don't cut off salt completely from your diet because this might cause Keto flu symptoms that some people have experience. Also, don't try to modify the diet on your own and add fruit or vegetables just because you have been told they are healthy. If you want to see real results from the carnivore diet, you need to ensure that you follow it properly. Another common mistake is to avoid fatty meat because of reasons like cholesterol. Fatty meat is recommended on a diet and will provide your body with good cholesterol. As long as you avoid these kinds of mistakes, the diet should work well for you.

Take Support

If you find this diet or any diet tough to follow or are struggling through it, reach out for support. Don't try to go through it alone. Everyone knows how hard it can be to break any habit or create new ones. The journey of weight loss, in particular, can be a very frustrating one. In such times, find a source of support like family or friends whom you are comfortable with. If not, there are a lot of support groups online as well that can help you. Do whatever it takes to keep yourself healthy and happy. A lot of the forums on carnivore dieting will help you meet other people just like you who can help you out.

Deciding on Long-Term or Short-Term

You might be wondering if the diet is safe to follow in the long term. The carnivore diet is usually used by people on a short-term basis to help them lose weight; however, if you take a look at online forums and testimonials, you find that many people have followed the diet for years on end and lived a healthy life. There are always exceptions to the rule, and some health conditions might be a problem, so consult your doctor to find out if you can follow this meat-centric diet safely for longer than you originally planned.

Optimizing the Carnivore Diet

Any diet could be customized for an individual and for their intended purpose. The following tips will help you in optimizing the diet for yourself if you want to lose weight while getting healthy.

Eat eggs

Try and add eggs to your diet although it is an all meat diet. Eggs are allowed, and we recommend it. They contain a lot of necessary nutrients that will benefit your body. So cook eggs in different ways and try and add them to your diet once in a while.

Eat offal

A lot of people usually overlook offal and avoid its consumption; however, trust us when we say that it is beneficial for your health. Offal like the liver is very rich in vital nutrients such as folate, vitamin A, choline and iron. Eating animal liver is like taking a natural multivitamin for your body. You can also eat fish liver, which is a good source of both vitamin D and B12.

More seafood

Don't just eat red meat. The all meat diet includes seafood and recommends its consumption for better health. Seafood is a nutrient-rich addition to your carnivorous diet. They contain a lot of omega 3 fatty acids, iron, copper, manganese and vitamin D. Seafood is a rare source of selenium, which the diet of most people lacks but is good for health. The omega 3's from fish will particularly benefit your heart health. There are no restrictions on which seafood you should or should not eat so make them a regular part of your diet; however, just like meat, you should buy fish that has been freshly caught from the wild and not those sourced from fish farms. The latter is more likely to have been fed chemicals or hormones to grow faster, and these will also come into your diet. We do understand that some people have not had fish as a part of their diet before so we recommend that you try it for a while by eating different varieties and styles of cooking. For those who still prefer not to eat fish, various fish oil supplements will work well. Your end goal is to eat as many necessary nutrients as possible to optimize your health while on the carnivore diet.

Intermittent Fasting

Intermittent fasting is explained in detail in another section of the book. We highly recommend trying it along with the carnivore diet to see the best results. Fasting is not the same as a starvation diet and will benefit you in various ways. This technique will add further changes in the body along with the carnivore diet. Your growth hormone production will increase while blood sugar, as well as insulin, decreases. People generally opt to add intermittent fasting to their routine because it is ideal to fasten the process of weight loss. It will aid your metabolic system and has an enhancing effect on your immune system. Read the section on intermittent fasting to learn about it in detail.

Plant foods with zero-calories

Spices are a form of plant-sourced foods that have no calories in them. This is why they are in the grey area where the plant foods are concerned. These along with herbs can be used to enhance the taste of your meat-based diet. The herbs and spices have nutritional value that is added to your diet. A variety of herbs like rosemary are even used as medicinal supplements.

Good quality meat

Even if the diet is meat based, quality matters. Eating just any random meat product will not be ideal for your health. Sourcing the best quality of meat will help your purpose.

Grass-fed meat or pastured meat is much better than any meat from factory farmed animals. The latter are fed hormones or chemicals that accumulate in your body and harm you in the long run. The principle is the same for seafood, which should be caught fresh and not from fisheries.

Bone Broth

Like we mentioned before, among liquids, bone broth is one of the forms allowed other than water. Adding bone broth to your diet will have various benefits. It is an excellent source of collagen, which is necessary for good skin and bone health.

Before you start following the carnivore diet, get your blood tested. Repeat this after a few weeks of following the diet. It will help you in measuring the effect it is having on your body. You need to take note of changes in weight, energy level and even your digestive functions. The first week of adaptation might be a little hard, as there is a lot of fluctuation in your energy and appetite and you might find it difficult to concentrate as well. Try to take a week off work or start on a week when the workload is less.

How to Stay on Track on the Carnivore Diet

Here will give you some tips to help you stay on track while following the carnivore diet. We know how hard it can be to suddenly place restrictions on food and your usual lifestyle. This is why it can be too much for some people to stay on track and they end up failing to achieve their goals. You might feel like quitting or just lose focus at some point. This is why the following strategies will help you in your journey.

Visualize

Visualization can be a very effective mental strategy. When you want to see some positive changes in yourself and your life, visualize it happening. You need to imagine yourself kicking off your unhealthy dietary habits and staring the carnivore diet successfully. Picture how you want to look in a year or so and how you want to feel. This imagery should help you stay motivated until you manage to achieve it. You can even imagine yourself in a dress that doesn't fit you right now but looks stunning in the near future.

Be realistic

Expectations should always be attainable and realistic. When you set unrealistic expectations for yourself, you are setting yourself up for disappointment and failure. If you want to lose weight, think of a healthy goal for each month. A few pounds in a month is a healthy and attainable goal. But if you think you will lose 10 pounds in a couple of months, it is probably unrealistic. Manageable goals are easier to attain and in a healthy way.

Short-term goals

A lot of people don't realize the importance of short-term goals. It is not just about a long-term plan or an end result. Some small steps at a time will help you get further in your journey. They can be anything like a small habit that you want to kick off in that month. Ultimately, one by one you can kick off any bad habit and reach the optimal health you want to achieve. In one month, you can try to focus on eating on time and the next you can start adding exercise to your everyday routine. All of this is a way to get better in the long run.

CHAPTER SEVEN -

INTERMITTENT FASTING

If you want to lose weight while following the carnivore diet, you should also try implementing intermittent fasting in your routine. Fasting is a practice that has been practiced since ancient times in various cultures around the world. Don't mistake fasting with starving though. Intermittent fasting does not work like some fad diet that tells you to starve yourself for a week to lose five pounds. The latter is a completely unreasonable practice that will have a negative impact on your health. Intermittent fasting, on the other hand, is beneficial for your health and is a recommended addition to your diet to just aid in the process of losing weight.

Intermittent fasting is a unique and effective way to increase the effectiveness of the carnivore diet both in terms of weight and health benefits. The protocol is quite simple, but it is true that not everyone can follow it. But the benefits will probably prompt you to at least try; however, we think that you should do this only after the first month or so of beginning the carnivore diet. The initial phase will already be a drastic change that you need to get adapted to. If you try and tinker with the diet in this initial phase, it will get much more difficult for you. So once this phase has passed, try intermittent fasting.

First, you have to understand what intermittent fasting is. It is a technique where you follow a diet with periods in between where no eating is allowed. These could be a no-food period of anything between 15 to 24 hours in a day. But you are allowed to fast more than a day at a time. This is how it is different from a starvation diet or some unhealthy fad diet. You are just taught how you restrain from eating and observe a fast period every few days in a week. It might sound hard right now, especially if you have never fasted before, but it is not. A lot of people have tried intermittent fasting to lose weight and for its various health benefits. They have found it effective, and we recommend it along with the carnivore diet to aid you more efficiently. You will be able to lose weight much faster, improve your metabolism, gain muscle and then maintain a healthy weight.

Intermittent fasting is a flexible plan that can be adjusted according to one's health and needs. It can vary from person to person so you can implement a fasting plan according to your ability. While the carnivore diet is more focused on what you eat, intermittent fasting helps you in controlling how much food you eat. This way you exercise control over the quality as well as the quantity of food. Most of us have an unhealthy habit of eating at the wrong time and overeating after missing timely meals. The intermittent fasting plan helps to exercise more discipline with regard to this. It can be very helpful for those who have a bad habit of giving in to cravings or overeating. When you have restricted eating periods on your diet, you will automatically be eating lesser, so you will see faster results than just following the carnivore diet.

According to the type of lifestyle you lead, you can choose a different method of intermittent fasting. Having a diet suited personally to you will help you in following through with it. A lot of people don't realize how important it is to pay attention to their individual needs. You cannot expect the same plan that worked for someone else to always work for you. This is why there are different types of intermittent fasting that we allow you to choose from. In fact, in some of these, you are even allowed to eat although in limited quantities.

Lean Gain Method

One of the methods of intermittent fasting is the lean gain diet. In this type, you are allowed to eat for 8 hours in the day while the rest of the 16 hours have to be a fasting period. There is no specification given for timings in the day so you can adjust this according to your schedule. All you need to ensure is no food in the fasting period. Your food can also be adjusted accordingly. If you exercise a lot on a particular day, you can add more fat to the meal. On a more sedentary day opt for more protein and limit the fat. This helps you maintain a healthy balance.

WEEKLY METHOD

In this type of intermittent fasting, you just have to fast for one day in the week. This means a 24-hour fast in a seven-day week. The rest of the six days will be the usual carnivore diet plan. Again, there are no timings that are specified. You can start in the morning if you want or even after lunch. Just ensure a 24-hour fast from that time. This is one of the easier types to follow and can be tried by beginners. This one-day fast acts as a boost to your healthy dietary change.

Alternate Day Method

This is another type of intermittent fasting but does not ask you to omit food at any point completely. Instead, you are supposed to eat normally on one day while the following day should involve minimal eating. This process should continue as every alternate day of minimal eating. On these days, you should focus on consuming half of what you usually eat. You should not focus on filling your stomach like you usually do and just eat a little bit that is enough. Don't try to overeat on the next day to make up for your day of less food.

Warrior Method

The warrior method is easy and quite popular. In this type of intermittent fasting, you have to fast for about 20 hours a day with 4 hours free to eat as you please. Don't be put off by the idea of the 20-hour fasting period because the warrior method allows you to eat a little even in those hours but very minimally. It is also recommended to eat more at night instead of the day.

If you find all these types of fasts complicated, just try practicing a little fasting once in a while. You can start by placing a restriction on food for a 15-hour period on the first day. Start with your fast in the morning and when you break your fast have a meal and sleep. This way you won't go to sleep hungry, and it will be easier for you. You can do this once a week if it is hard for you. Then you can try it again after two days of normal eating. This way you can try about three days of intermittent fasting in a week later; however, make sure you don't fast continuously for two days at a time or more than 3-4 days in a week. The first few days that you try intermittent fasting might be difficult for you. There is an adaptation period that will take a few days. Give yourself a chance to get past this initial phase, and you will find it much easier. Be easy on yourself and don't try to impose strict restrictions in the beginning. Your body is already going through a change with the carnivore diet so it will cause unwanted stress. Also, don't try to use this as an excuse to starve yourself because you think it will help you get thin faster. Not providing your body with adequate food will only do you harm. Instead, follow a healthy plan of intermittent fasting once in a while with your carnivore diet.

Tips to aid in intermittent fasting:

- Eat a sufficient amount of the foods allowed on the carnivore diet when it is not a fasting day. Don't overeat to compensate for fasting but don't eat too little either. It will just make it harder for you when you are practicing fasting.

- If you feel hungry on a no food period, try drinking some green tea. This will help to curb hunger pangs. Don't add any sweetener to it. Drinking black coffee will also give your body a boost.

- Remember to stay hydrated whether it is a fasting day or not. Dehydration on a fasting day, in particular, can be very harmful to your health. Keep some water at hand at all times. If you feel nauseous or weak, you can even add some electrolytes.

- Eat healthy dietary fat sources as recommended on the carnivore diet. Butter or eggs are not your enemy and will benefit you.

Benefits of intermittent fasting:

Weight loss

The main aim behind trying intermittent fasting is usually to aid in weight loss. Thankfully, it fulfills the purpose and is not a wasted effort at all. It reduces your intake of food, which in turn means you are consuming fewer calories; however, this will not hold true if you try to make up for a fasting day by overeating on the other days. It also enhances the functioning of the hormones, which facilitate weight loss. Since levels of insulin reduce with an increase in nor-adrenaline and growth hormone, fat molecules break down further. Calorie consumption is reduced while metabolic activity is optimized. One of the best parts is that it particularly helps to lose weight from the belly that can otherwise be tough.

Insulin resistance is reduced

Intermittent fasting on the carnivore diet will benefit people who are at risk of or suffering from diabetes type 2. If a person has diabetes type 2, their blood sugar level is high, and the resistance to insulin in their body increases. This can be very harmful to health and cause further ailments. Intermittent fasting has been known to help to reduce blood sugar levels along with reducing the resistance to insulin.

Reduced inflammation

If your body suffers from a lot of oxidative stress, it will increase the rate of aging and also increase the risk of various chronic ailments. This oxidative stress is caused by unstable molecules reacting with stable molecules of protein or DNA. This then damages the good molecules and harms your body. Including intermittent fasting will help to improve the resistance of your body to such conditions.

Improved heart condition

Heart disease has increased alarmingly over the last few decades. A bad diet is one of the main causes of this. High blood pressure, bad cholesterol, high levels of triglycerides and high blood sugar increase the risk of heart diseases; however, intermittent fasting helps to reduce the risk associated with all of these and thus improve heart health.

Functioning of cells

Food plays many different roles in your body. If you don't eat enough during a particular period, it will prompt the cells in the body to start repairing or regenerating. The hormonal levels in your body will change, and they will work to make your body burn fat for energy as well. The drop-in insulin level also facilitates this process of burning fat. Instead, there will be an increase in the growth hormone in the body too. The composition of genes and molecules that support a long healthy life will see a positive change. This will also improve your immune system. During the fasting process, cells also start removing wastes. Dysfunctional cells and proteins are broken down during a process known as autophagy. When autophagy increases, it has been known to reduce the risk of diseases like cancer and Alzheimer's. The removal of waste build-up in cells is facilitated.

CHAPTER EIGHT -

CARNIVORE DIET FOOD LIST –
BREAKFAST, LUNCH, AND DINNER

The basic guideline for the carnivore diet is to eat meat and sometimes, other animal-sourced food. There is no other rule to this diet that you need to concern yourself with. It doesn't matter what time you eat, how much you eat, what your portion size is or even what the percentage of your macronutrients are. Just eat when you feel hungry and only eat meat. In this section, we will clarify any doubts about what you can eat and also help you get an understanding of how you can plan your breakfast lunch or dinner according to the carnivore diet.

Meat

The usual food source in this diet is meat from various animals. You can eat red meat like beef, pork, wild game, lamb or even the meat of birds. Out if all meat options on this diet, beef is the most recommended one. You can also eat white meat from chicken or turkey. This also includes fish or any seafood like fresh oysters, lobster, crab, shrimp and squid. Organ meat is also allowed so you can eat the liver, bone marrow, heart, brain or kidney for any animal. Eggs are also a good source of protein on this diet and can be sourced from chickens, geese or ducks. Don't try to eat only lean meat, include the fatty cuts in your diet too. The fat from the meat provides your daily nutritional requirements. It will also provide you with the required protein, minerals and other nutrients. The fatty cut of meat will help to make your diet more palatable.

Among the meat options you have, we will give you the best cuts and types to choose from. If you like lamb, you can eat lamb chops, ribs or shank. For poultry, wings, thighs and drumsticks are good. In case of pork, opt for meat from the shoulder, ribs, butt roast or pork belly. Fish gives you many options like salmon, shrimp, trout, scallops, sardines, mackerel and crab. You can also have bone broth from any of the animals.

You might wonder if it is necessary only to eat grass-fed meat. While this would be the healthiest option for you, it is understandable that it is also more expensive. Don't let this bother you too much and opt for meats that fall within your budget. The high cost of grass-fed meat should not stop you from beginning the carnivore diet. When it comes to processed meat, at least avoid these on the first 30 days of trying the carnivore diet. This will allow the diet to be more effective and healthier for you. You can eat bacon but avoid sausages.

Organ meat is recommended in the carnivore diet because they contain DHA and this will help to improve the functioning of the brain. It is a personal choice to include or omit offal from your diet.

Dairy

Certain foods are on the list that comes in the category of "maybe." You can have these in minimal amounts on occasion but not on a regular basis or in large amounts. These are technically animal sourced, so they don't completely defy the guidelines, but they are still not meat. These include dairy products like heavy cream, butter, ghee, milk, yogurt and cheese; however, most people prefer not to consume dairy especially if they want to lose weight faster. This is primarily because dairy contains lactose and even if it is consumed, should be minimal.

Water, tea and coffee

Water is your recommended beverage and should be preferred over anything else to stay hydrated no matter what diet you follow. Coffee and tea are exceptions to the restrictions on a diet despite being plant-sourced. The only rule is to have them black and without any sugar or additives. These two ingredients actually have a lot of benefits by themselves and also work as a natural insecticide. It can be hard for people to adapt to the carnivore diet if they also have to adapt to caffeine withdrawal at the same time; however, once you get adapted to the diet, try to cut the caffeine habit too.

Salt and pepper are the only taste enhancers allowed, and these should also be used within a limit. Spices are actually another exception to the rule that is not stressed on much. It is recommended to omit these from the diet as well, but you can choose to use some for added flavor in your food. Just try not to over-do it. Turmeric is one of the beneficial spices that should be considered since it aids in immunity and also improves cognitive and brain health. Cayenne pepper has particular benefits in the process of weight loss.

Herbs

Herbs are not only flavorful but also have numerous health benefits. Adding some of these to your meat-based meals will help to improve your health and also add a variety of taste to this restrictive diet. Cinnamon is one such beneficial herb that adds flavor and also regulates blood sugar levels. It actually acts like a type of natural insulin. Another herb that is infused with flavor is oregano. It contains many antioxidants and blends well with different flavors. Rosemary should also be considered since it is helpful in alleviating inflammation in your body. Inflammation is one of the main causes of arthritis and rosemary can reduce the associated risk. Thyme is rich in antioxidants and is useful for maintaining a healthy respiratory system.

Supplements

Usually, you wouldn't need any extra supplements; however, some people do require them, and these can be had during the adaptation period. The permitted supplements include Himalayan salt, electrolytes and lipase or Ox bile for GI support; however, after the adaptation period passes, cut these off.

Let's see what a day on the carnivore diet will look like in terms of your meals.

Breakfast

In the morning you can eat a few eggs that can be boiled or cooked in butter. You can also add cheese and ham to this meal. If you want tea or coffee, make it black.

Lunch

In the afternoon, go ahead and eat a rib eye steak. You can also have other beef cuts like sirloin, strip or chuck eye. If you don't want a steak, opt for a roast. This will seem like a dream come true for those who previously had to avoid this on another diet.

Dinner

Your dinner can be a hamburger patty with some cooked bacon. You can even have an extra patty if the lack of buns makes you feel dissatisfied. You can also opt for a T-bone steak instead of the patties.

We recommend abstaining from snacks, and this is easy because meat is very filling. It keeps you much more satisfied, and you will rarely feel hungry until it is time for your next meal. If you still feel hungry all the time, you should consider increasing the fatty cuts in your meals, as these are more filling. When you absolutely must snack, try some pork rinds.

Foods to avoid while on the Carnivore Diet

On the carnivore diet, you nearly have to stop eating everything that does not fall in the category of meat.

- Vegetables

- Fruit

- Nuts

- Seeds

- Legumes

- Grains

- Pasta

- Bread

- Seasonings or sauces

- Alcohol

- Processed meat

- Processed food of any type

- No vegetable oils

Avoid any processed meats like ham, salami, pepperoni or chorizo. These are the carbohydrate fillers, which should be avoided especially on this diet; however, if you can stick to the best diet possible in the first month, later these processed meats can sometimes be eaten as snacks. When you are traveling these might be your best option to stick to the diet; however, try to avoid anything processed as much as possible.

Also, avoid buying pre-made sausages. These usually contain wheat, which is added to fill the sausage out. You can try making your own healthy ones at home. Don't buy cheap sausages on the market or hotdogs off the stand. These will affect your diet and can cause weight gain too.

CHAPTER NINE -

ADVANTAGE/DISADVANTAGE OF THE CARNIVORE DIET

In this section, we will take a look at some of the pros and cons of following this diet. Like everything else or any other diet, it has its own advantage and disadvantage.

Disadvantages of the Carnivore Diet

One of the disadvantages of an all meat diet is that it can harm your health instead of improving it if you don't eat meat that is of good quality. The cheaper industrially processed meat is usually full of many preservatives, residues and chemicals. These animals are fed food that is low quality and filled with toxins like pesticides, GMOs, antibiotics, etc. which then go into their body. You will thus be indirectly eating all these from the low-quality meat as well. This is why it is important to find meat from animals that are raised in pastures, grass-fed or fed organic food. This will ensure the animals were healthy, and so is the meat. This factor is essential when you follow a meat-based diet.

Since meat contains a lot of saturated fat and cholesterol, you will get a lot of it in your diet on a regular basis. This might be a disadvantage. The Trans fat from this diet might also prompt the liver to produce more cholesterol than required.

This is why you need to control the amount of fatty meat you consume regularly.

Another back draw is the high amount of sodium that is found in processed meat or salt-cured meat. Excessive consumption of sodium can escalate the risk of heart diseases or strokes and even be a problem for kidney function. This is why it is recommended to avoid processed meat like salami, jerky or ham in order to avoid the sodium excess. Fresh meat will have much lower levels of sodium and is not a cause for concern.

If you consider the cost factor, it is true that a meat diet is more expensive than a plant-based diet. The diet can be quite expensive if you are providing it not just for yourself but your entire family. Buying meat is expensive on a daily basis, especially if you want the good quality kind. Unless you have your own farm animals or can somehow process the meat yourself, you should be prepared to increase expenditure on food in your budget. One tip that will help is buying in bulk as it usually reduces the cost.

Advantages of the Carnivore Diet

The advantage of this diet is that it is fairly simple. It saves you a lot of time and energy since your ingredients and cooking process are both simplified. You won't just see improvement in your health but also notice that you spend a lot less of your day in the kitchen preparing food. Most of the cutting, processing, cooking parts involved in your usual day are removed when you follow the carnivore diet.

The carnivore diet is a great source of protein for the body. Protein is essential for maintaining many processed in the body to keep it healthy. This is why it is considered a building block of life. Since you will only be eating meat, you have a constant source of good protein for your body. Even a small amount of meat is densely packed with protein and will make up for the recommended daily allowance for a person. You will also be getting all the essential amino acids required by your body. Nine amino acids exist that cannot be made by the body even though they are essential for health. The proteins in meat contain amino acids and actually have all nine of them. This is why animal meat is considered a complete source of protein and supplements the body with these essential amino acids through the diet. In order for maintaining healthy bones, muscle and skin, these amino acids need to be provided regularly.

You will also e getting a good source of B-complex vitamins such as niacin, riboflavin, thiamine and vitamin B12. Meat contains all of these and thus helps to maintain energy levels and contributing to growth. These vitamins also help in better iron absorption. Meat will also provide other minerals such as zinc and selenium to your body.

Another advantage is that this diet has helped a lot of people overcome some chronic illnesses, which they could not otherwise treat. This includes autoimmune diseases and even includes Lyme disease. When other treatments and even a good doctor's protocol failed, this diet helped a lot of people get healthier on a purely meat-based diet.

CHAPTER TEN -

DIFFERENCE BETWEEN KETO DIET, PALEO DIET AND CARNIVORE DIET

As you know, the carnivore diet is often compared to the low carb and keto diet; however, the overlap with similarities between these diets ends at a certain point.

First, let's take a look at what each of these diets entail.

The Paleo Diet

In a nutshell, this diet says that if there is any food that a caveman did not eat, you should not eat it either. If you decide to follow the Paleo diet, you are allowed to eat anything that cave dwellers could hunt or gather and thus consume in their diet. This will include meat, nuts, fish, seeds, leafy greens and vegetables that grew regionally. You will have to give up all the processed food that is a part of the modern-day diet. This means the pasta, candy, cereals, etc. have to go. This diet does not tell you how much you should eat and does not set any calorie limitation for the day either. Instead, it is focused on improving the kind of food that you eat.

The Ketogenic Diet

The Keto diet is basically low carb and high-fat diet that allows moderate consumption of proteins. It is actually quite similar to other low carb diets like the Atkins diet. The intention of this diet is to eat a lot of fat and put your body in a constant state of ketosis. This ketosis process will push your body to burn the stored fat in your body as a source of energy. Instead of glucose, your body will turn to ketones. The diet pushes your metabolic system away from its dependence on carbs towards ketones and fat instead. There are a few versions of the Keto diet that can be adjusted to suit the person's level of activity in a day.

The Carnivore Diet

The carnivore diet is not about macros and is totally focused on one food: meat. In this diet, you are basically supposed to eat meat for all your meals and no other foods. The only exception if freshly sourced dairy products in a limited amount.

When it comes to weight loss, most recommended diets would tell you to consume a lower amount of carbs. The Keto diet reduces your carb intake while the carnivore diet completely removes carbs from your diet. How do you decide which is better? The Paleo diet advocates plant-based foods but don't these contain toxins and irritants like gluten? Then does it mean that the carnivore diet is the best option with only meat? There are groups of people who agree with this last synopsis while there are others who are completely against it; however, you are probably in the middle since you can see that the carnivore diet has its own unique benefits and can help you get lean and healthy.

The carbohydrate restrictions of the carnivore diet are actually much more extensive than what you see while following a low carb Keto diet. The Keto diet has a moderate amount of proteins with a high amount of fats and a small number of carbs. In the case of the carnivore diet, you will mostly be consuming proteins and fats almost exclusively.

Compared to the Keto diet, there has not been a much extensive study on the carnivore diet. The Keto diet has been researched for a long time and thus has a lot of scientific backing; however, the same work has not been put into understanding the carnivore diet. This is why there is no such exact ratio to guide you on how much fat and protein you should consume on the carnivore diet. On the other hand, the Keto diet usually has a standard ratio to dictate the number of fats, protein and carbs you need to consume on a daily basis. In a Keto diet, the standard ratio is 60-70% of fats, 20-30% of proteins and 5-10 % of carbohydrates. The carnivore diet allows you to eat without any macronutrient guideline.

In the carnivore diet, the only time carbs are allowed if it comes in the form of fresh dairy products. There are certain dairy products which are fresh or fermented that contain carbs in a decent amount. While this source of carbs is allowed on the carnivore diet, there are many who don't even consume this. In a Keto diet, you are allowed to have low carb vegetables, but this is not allowed on the carnivore diet; however, we recommend that you follow a healthier approach that balances the amount of meat you consume with some animal products like eggs or milk. This will help in a healthier approach to the carnivore diet.

The Paleo and Keto diet allow a certain number of spices, salt, oils, etc. that help to add value as well as taste to your meals; however, in the carnivore diet, it is slightly debatable whether these are allowed or not. These ingredients are sourced from plants and the carnivore diet emphasizes eating only animal-sourced food.

The Ketogenic diet is a low carb diet while the carnivore diet eliminated carbs completely. This is why the latter is considered much more restrictive than Keto. You can also eat plant foods in the Keto diet, and this includes nuts and seeds. Unlike Keto, all of this is restricted in the carnivore diet. On the other hand, some high carb foods are restricted on the Keto diet, but these are allowed on the carnivore diet as long as they have been taken from an animal source. The amount of carbs in the food is not of consequence since these dairy foods are to be consumed minimally anyhow.

Compared to the other two diets, people usually follow the carnivore diet as a last resort. This diet is often taken up when the other diets don't work or give efficient results. People who suffer from health issues like chronic pain or digestive issues also try the carnivore diet to see if it will help to alleviate these problems. After someone has tried Paleo, Keto, intermittent fasting and many other diets, they are finally open to trying a more extreme diet like this all meat one; however, just like other diets, it will work for some and not so much for others.

CHAPTER ELEVEN -

WHO SHOULD FOLLOW CARNIVORE DIET?

You may be wondering if this meat-centric diet is appropriate for you or not. We recommend that you try it with some exceptions to the rule. In this section, you will learn more about who will benefit from this diet and who should not follow it. Before you go into the diet and eliminate all other food, you should consult a doctor or dietician who will check your health issues and medical background to determine what is appropriate for you. Every individual can have a plan that is optimized to suit his or her specific needs.

The carnivore diet is usually recommended more often for those who suffer from certain food intolerances. The diet is prescribed on a short-term basis for such people to help them find what foods are actually aggravating their condition. You can slowly introduce new foods into your diet and keep checking which has a negative impact on your health. Many people have found the diet useful in this respect. Food intolerance is suffered by a lot of people, and they find the carnivore diet useful in eliminating the negative symptoms associated with it.

The intolerance is a negative reaction that takes place when the person eats a particular food or even a food group. Some of the most common food intolerances are caused by wheat or dairy products. This will mean that such people have intolerance to a substance in those foods like gluten or lactose. Thus, they can prevent the symptoms by eliminating these foods. Other ingredients that might cause an issue are lectin or phytic acid that is usually found in plant foods. These ingredients can cause an issue with digestion; however, the carnivore diet doesn't contain them so you can identify which food is causing the issue excluding the meat that you eat. Likewise, you will eliminate all potential intolerance causing foods and then slowly re-introduce them one at a time. As you observe the reaction your body has to each food, you will know which to eliminate from the diet.

If you have high blood pressure, you might really want to try the carnivore diet. We will give you an old account of the proof that this diet aids in maintaining better blood pressure levels. Like we told you before, the Inuit people of Greenland were originally following a diet that was carnivorous in nature. They ate a lot of meat and fish and very little fruit or vegetables. Their diet was quite high in animal fat; however, at some point around the late 1900s, a few of these families decided to immigrate to Denmark. When they migrated, they were introduced to a more modern Danish diet, which consisted of more plant-based foods and dairy products. Their meat intake and the animal-sourced foods in their diet were greatly reduced. When research was done, it showed that this change in their diet actually raised their blood pressure by more than ten points compared to before. They followed the guidelines that we are all still fed about a healthy diet when they moved to Denmark; however, this proved that the reduction of meat did not actually benefit their blood pressure but raised it to an unhealthy level. Even among the Masai of Africa, research showed that only 1% of the men who followed the meat diet suffered from high blood pressure. Barely any of them had any issues throughout their life, and the blood pressure points only increased a little when they crossed the age of 60. This is why we recommend that you try eating in the old Inuit or Masai tribe way to try and improve your blood pressure levels as well.

The carnivore diet can also be very beneficial for those who suffer from obesity or are overweight to an unhealthy extent. Obesity is actually a very modern-day disease. If you look back in history, even among your own ancestors, there was barely any mention of people being so overweight. The main cause behind this weight-related disease is the modern-day diet and the negative impact the food industry has had on it. Let us consider the people of Masai or Samburu. Obesity did not even exist among these people when they followed the all-meat diet.

All these people had an appropriate body weight, and this was stable throughout their lives. You might argue that you can see the Eskimos who follow the all-meat diet and they look fat; however, this is not true. Their features are healthy in peculiarity of their race. It has nothing to do with being over-weight or corpulent. They look a little healthier due to their puffy warm garments that are required to shield their bodies from the cold. When you see them without these bulky clothing, we assure you that there are no unhealthy abdominal folds or bulging tummies. These people don't have some immunity to being fat but are just healthier because of the very diet they follow.

If they were to move to a city with access to modern foods, they would get fat just as quickly as anyone else. Considering these instances, you can see why we recommend the carnivore diet for people who suffer from obesity. It can be hard for obese people to follow other strict diets that require them to measure their portions or count their calories on a regular basis. It often leaves them frustrated and hungry. Ultimately, the diet is usually too hard for most to follow through with; however, the carnivore diet makes things much simpler and is easy to follow in the long term. The person is also allowed to eat as much as they need to satisfy their hunger; however, it still helps to lose a lot of the unhealthy fats from the body. So if you want to lose weight, try the carnivore diet for a few months at least.

The carnivore diet will also benefit those with a higher risk of heart diseases. Like we mentioned in a previous chapter, this particular benefit of the diet was proven when there was a study done on the people of Point Hope in Alaska. The people of that region were largely untouched by the unhealthy modern diet and continued to follow the Eskimo diet of meat or fish. The study showed that compared to the population of the rest of the places in the US, the incidence of cardiovascular issues was nearly ten times lower. Their triglyceride levels were also much healthier at an average of 85 mg/dL while the rest had an average above 100mg/dL. If your family history or your personal health puts you at a higher risk of heart diseases, you can try to reduce the chances by following this meat-centric diet.

Who should not try it?

First off, we don't recommend the carnivore diet or any other strict diet for people who suffer from eating disorders. In case you have suffered from anorexia, bulimia or any such disorders, consult a professional to get a healthy diet that will help you heal. Your personal health has to be your priority and not your weight. You need to make more of an effort to instill body positivity. Once your doctor says you are at a healthy point and can try the diet, go ahead. But do not try it without proper consultation.

The carnivore diet is also not suitable for people who suffer from any severe kidney diseases. If you already suffer from some serious issue with your kidney or any other organ, your doctor will guide you with the best possible diet. For those who have a healthy kidney function, the diet can actually aid in improving functioning since it helps to get rid of excess glucose while insulin sensitivity is improved.

Athletes and sportspersons may also wonder if they should follow the carnivore diet. There are no adequate studies that can exactly dictate this. There are a lot of followers of the carnivore diet who claim that their strength improved on the diet. However, it takes time for the body to get used to using meat for energy. The diet is usually not recommended for athletes since they require a high amount of energy on a constant basis. A low carb diet like the Ketogenic diet can be adjusted for their needs, but the carnivore diet is much more restrictive and might not be appropriate.

If you are wondering if the diet is safe to follow, we will reply in the affirmative subject to the same conditions of any other diet. Some people react better to certain diets while others will react differently. For most people who have tried it, it has proven to be safe and effective. You already know that it is not animal fat but sugar that is the main cause of increased heart diseases so you should not worry about this aspect either; however, there have not been any long-term studies done on this diet, so you won't find any concrete evidence to prove it safe or unsafe.

CHAPTER TWELVE -

WHY PLANTS ARE ELIMINATED ON THE CARNIVORE DIET

You might be curious about the reasoning behind eliminating all plant foods from your diet. For years you have probably heard that a plant-based diet is your healthiest choice and also the best bet to lose weight. The common belief is that the more fruit and vegetables you eat, the healthier you will be; however, were you aware of the fact that nearly all the junk food that you eat is plant-based? Trust us when we say this because it is true. Do you still believe that all plant-based foods are healthy? We aren't disregarding the fact that a plant-based diet works quite well for some people, but it is not the case for some others.

Every individual has a different and unique genetic makeup, immune system and microbiome scheme. The basic biology is the same, so everyone assumes that what works for one person will also work for the other; however, the biochemical makeup is completely different and not the same as the basic anatomy. The plant foods that you eat could be a cause for inflammation, digestive issues and even hormonal imbalance in your body. If you suffer from metabolic issues or a leaky gut, this can also be due to the so-called "good" foods sourced from plants. This is why it is not appropriate to make a generic statement that plant foods are good for everyone. Such generalization can be misleading and even harmful for people who are actually affected negatively by plant compounds.

There are a lot of diets out there that people follow randomly without doing due research. Most of these recommend the elimination of fats or carbs and ask you to eat as many fruit or vegetables as possible. One such type of fad diet involves a cleaning process, which is done by only drinking green smoothies. You are supposed to eat no solid foods and only blend all green ingredients into a smoothie as your meal substitute. There was an instance of a woman following this diet that was published in a prominent American medical journal. This woman ended up developing acute kidney failure thanks to this diet. We aren't trying to prove that green vegetables are all harmful. You don't even have to stop drinking green smoothies; however, the point is that while such a diet might have been helpful for one person who recommended it to that woman, it had a very negative impact on her life. Any food can have an opposite effect on the body of one person even if it has a positive effect on another.

In such cases, it may be hard to identify what exactly is causing an unwanted symptom in your body. If you eat a variety of foods in your diet, it is hard to pinpoint the particular aggravator. It might just be one specific type of vegetable that is harmful to you. In order to identify these, a lot of people have used the carnivorous diet as an aid. Not only does it help to find the perpetrator, but an all meat diet has also been helpful in reversing health issues. The carnivore diet has also helped in restoring hormonal balance for a more stable system. This is why we are trying to explain why going all meat will benefit you and why plants are not always are great as they are made out to be.

Among the majority of vegetarians, they always have arguments to rationalize why they choose not to eat meat and why others should do the same. One such argument is that eating meat is a form of animal cruelty and this applies to using any animal related products as well. All living creatures have an equal right to live and killing them for food is a violation of this right. They all say that if everyone stopped eating meat, all animals could live peacefully and rightfully and this would make the world a better place; however, if you use the living creature argument, you have to consider that all plants are living beings as well. Why do animals have a greater right to live than plants? In fact, plants should be spared since they cannot defend themselves in any way. Animals, on the other hand, have their own ways of defending themselves from other predators as well as humans. The only way that plants can defend themselves is when you consume them. This is when their compounds will react with your body and cause inflammation, autoimmune disorders, pain and some can even cause death. We all know that there are certain types of plants that can be poisonous if ingested.

Plants can produce a number of toxins or anti-nutrients that will harm your body. A lot of people are completely clueless about this negative aspect and only focus on how many nutrients a plant has or what its benefits are. Among plants that cause inflammation, you would be surprised to learn that it includes commonly consumed ones like tomato, potato, eggplant, and even the goji berry. Seeds are considered super food, but they usually contain phytic acid, which is an anti-nutrient. This phytic acid is also found in grains and legumes. It affects the absorption of minerals like zinc, iron, and calcium in the body. Green leafy vegetables are also commonly encouraged in a healthy diet as superfoods, but they contain oxalate that some bodies cannot process. If the oxalate is not digested, it can be a cause of oxidative stress and chronic pain. The lectin in grains and legumes can also be a cause for health issues. This ingredient causes leaky gut, autoimmune conditions and also increases inflammation. Lectin also alters the microbiome system in your body.

When plants are being grown, a lot of insecticides, pesticides, etc. are used to help in the process. These chemical substances contain salicylates that build up in the human body over time. High level of this compound in the body is a cause of ulcers and tinnitus. Usually, the main plant foods that increase salicylates in our body include grapes, avocados, honey, berries, dry fruit and even spices. Do you eat a lot of cruciferous vegetables such as broccoli, cabbage or kale? These are a common component in weight loss diets; however, they contain goitrogens that can be very harmful to the thyroid hormone level in your body.

As you can see, there are various harmful ingredients in different plants that can wreak havoc on your body. Many of these can cause some serious problems for your health and are obviously not healthy for you even if they are for someone else. Don't think that all plants are bad for everyone and that they should be eliminated from your diet forever; however, you have to be aware of the fact that everything has its good and bad side. This applies to plant foods like anything else. Don't assume that eating a lot of plants in your diet will ensure good health and longevity. It might for some and will not for others. All this information is probably removing your doubt about trying the carnivore diet by now. You can understand why there are benefits to removing plants from your diet and switching to an all meat diet at least for a short-term basis.

Going long term would depend on its effect on your body and your personal choice.

CHAPTER THIRTEEN -

MYTHS ABOUT MEAT

A lot of stigma has been attached to meat in the past few years. Many nutritionists advise people to quit eating meat or to reduce it from their diet. They should replace unhealthy meat with healthy green vegetables and fruit instead; however, do you still think you should? By now you have a good idea about why an all meat diet is recommended and why plants are eliminated from the diet. In this section, we will clarify some of the doubt you might have about following a completely meat-centric diet. Most of what you have heard is just a myth and does not have any scientific basis.

Meat is unhealthy

You have probably been among the people who were told to stop eating meat and eat plant foods instead. Meat is considered unhealthy and the cause of many health issues; however, this is not true. Meat is actually healthy food and has many benefits for your body. Despite this, a lot of misconceptions surround the consumption of meat. More and more people have started following a vegetarian or vegan diet, as they have been told that a diet that is plant-based is able to fulfill all the nutritional requirements of their body and while meat will not. If you study the diet of our ancestors, you can easily find out that meat was the main component of the human diet for a very long time. Grains and legumes were introduced in the human diet only when cultivation began around ten thousand years ago. Prior to this cultivation period, human survived on meat for millions of years. Doesn't this mean that the human body is much more accustomed to a meat-based diet? When the modern diet started relying on agricultural produce, it also saw a widespread increase in the incidence of health issues like diabetes, obesity, cardiovascular diseases and even osteoporosis. More people suffered from skin issues and inflammation. All of these were barely recorded before the change in the diet happened. When you compare the statistics of health conditions of these two periods with respect to the diets, it seems obvious that a meat-based diet is healthier. Human genes developed and evolved in the earlier era and had since only undergone a bare 0.02% change. This is why the human body is still more suited to function optimally on a diet that is filled with meat as the main source of food. Can you still label meat unhealthy?

Humans Aren't Meant to Eat Meat

Another common myth is that humans were not originally meant to eat meat at all; however, if you take a look at your body, you will understand that it was designed to aid in that very process. The molars and incisors in your dentition serve the purpose of tearing and grinding meat. If we weren't meant to eat any meat, our digestive system would not be able to digest it either. Instead, it would be more similar to herbivorous animals like cows that eat grass. But we know that our digestive system is much more complex and different than a cow. If we weren't meant to eat meat, our ancestors would have been constantly ill and barely managed to survive; however, this is not true either. In fact, they barely suffered from half of the ailments that the present generation has to deal with. The more likely chance is that humans were not meant to eat according to this agriculture-based diet, which has caused an increase in diseases and health issues.

Meat Causes High Blood Pressure

For some reason, meat is given a lot of blame for increasing blood pressure levels in the body; however, the truth is that meat helps to stabilize the level of blood sugar. A steady level has to be maintained in order to treat conditions like diabetes type 2. More meat in your diet will also help to stabilize your level of energy throughout the day and prevents energy drops that are experienced in a high carb diet.

Meat does not Provide Vitamins and Proteins

A lot of people say that you can afford to cut off meat from your diet because it doesn't really provide any essential nutrients or proteins to the body the way plants do. In reality, meat is an ideal source of good protein. No supplements will aid you in the growth or regeneration of muscle the way meat can. It is also a great source of minerals like iron and zinc. Meat will also provide your body with vitamins that promote good health like niacin and thiamine. All of these helps to improve your energy levels and aid in muscle repair as well. Your neurotransmitter health is also maintained with the help of the amino acids provided by the protein in meat. If you cut off meat from your diet, you will see a deficiency in these essential amino acids that cannot be internally produced by the body and have to be ingested from sources like meat. If there is an imbalance in amino acids, you will also see an increase in issues like anxiety and depression. A meat-centric diet aids in reducing such symptoms and maintains better mental health along with physical health.

It is quite clear that meat is unjustly given a bad name in the world of nutrition. Over the years, more and more diets have been developed without any scientific basis. Each of these will try to criminalize some particular type of food in order to promote its own benefits; however, most of these are completely pointless claims and will instead cause harm to your body. You can see that all the myths associated with meat are just misconceptions. You should not resist following the carnivore diet due to any such myths.

CHAPTER FOURTEEN -

HOW DOES A HIGH-FAT DIET BENEFIT YOU?

You might have noticed that the carnivore diet claims to help you lose weight but also advocates high-fat consumption. This can seem a contradictory system since fats are always blamed for obesity or excessive weight gain or any illnesses related to this; however, the carnivore diet, as well as the Ketogenic diet, works to debunk this myth. You don't have to cut off all fat from your diet just to lose weight or to be healthier. Carbohydrates are much worse for your health than fats. In this section, we will help you understand why we advocate a meat-centric diet that is high in fats.

History shows that our ancestors evolved with the help of a carbohydrate-free diet. They were hunters and gatherers and usually consumed meat for food. Their diet only consisted of food that could be easily accessed. Meat from animals or fish was easiest since they hunted them down. They also gathered other food to eat when there wasn't sufficient meat, but this was rare. In any case, their food was not starchy like the foods that the modern diet is comprised of. Do you think they ate any pasta or were able to bake bread? Even potatoes did not get included in the diet until the agricultural revolution. The last hundred years have made drastic changes in our diet, and we doubt that our genes have been able to adapt to this change. Our body is more attuned to eating how they ate for thousands of years at a time. This is why the processed foods of the industrial revolution don't add up to a healthy diet.

When all the factories started coming up everywhere, the food industry becomes much commercialized. Now you can see hundreds of food factories with thousands of products for you. It may seem like we are privileged to have so many options to eat from but it does not benefit our health in any way. Our modern-day diet is affected greatly by the propaganda of these companies to sell their product and earn a profit. They are not concerned with keeping you healthy and well but just want to sell more to earn more. These various processed foods on the shelves of grocery stores are nearly always packed with refined sugars, coloring and various additives that are not safe for your body. At a certain point, to sell their products to the health conscious, the industries started selling low-fat products. Fats were demonized and blamed for all weight-related issues in particular. Thus, people started blaming fats and tried to eliminate it from their diet. Even all the foods that are labeled low fat contain harmful processed ingredients that are not healthy for you. Since people started reducing fat consumption, the dependence on carbs in the diet went up. This high carbohydrate diet was the main reason that obesity became so prevalent in this generation. The high-fat diet of our ancestors did not make them over-weight and benefited their lifestyle.

You need to understand why fats are better than carbs. The carbohydrates in your diet are taken in and the body will break these into simple sugars. Since you eat more carbs, there is more sugar. The sugar goes into your bloodstream and the level of glucose spikes. To counteract against this spike in blood sugar, more insulin is produced in the body.

Insulin is a hormone that promotes the storage of fat instead of burning it. Therefore, the more sugar you eat, the more insulin is produced and the more fat is stored. You can see how easily you gain weight on a high carb diet due to this. During this time, your body will also start developing carvings for all these high carb or sugar-laden foods. It will constantly make you hungry and the process is repeated when you eat again. This is why it is important to restrict carbohydrate consumption more than fats. It will help to stabilize your blood sugar level and also regulate insulin production. When carbs are reduced, it will also push your body to start burning fats instead of storing it. Thus, the fats will become your source of energy and you will also lose weight.

The body usually finds it easier to burn carbs compared to fats. This is why glucose is always the first choice and during that time, fats are stored in the liver. But over time, this takes its toll on the liver and causes a fatty liver. There is a certain limit to how much fat the liver can store and remain healthy. On the modern diet, this limit is easily crossed. This is why it is important to restrict carbs so that the body has no option but to switch from glucose to fats as its main source of energy. The carnivore diet is a no- carb diet with high-fat content. This makes it much easier for your body to switch on the fat burning mode for more energy. Burning fats takes more time than burning carbs so you get a constant source of energy. Insulin production will also reduce to a more normal level and hunger pangs or carvings will slowly subside. Eating foods that have more dietary fats and no sugar will only benefit your health.

On a high carb diet, the body burns it as a primary source of energy; however, there is always some residue of fat in the cells from these carbohydrates. On the other hand, when fats are burned this does not happen. As you switch to the ketosis mode and burn more fat, glycation of proteins in the body reduces. Due to this, inflammation in the body will also reduce. When more fat is burned, more ketones are produced. Converting ketones to energy is a much easier process than the conversion of carbs to glycogen. Burning the stored and consumed fat will produce more energy in the body and also ensure that more energy is available to the body itself.

Like we mentioned before, ketosis is beneficial for brain health. The brain always prefers ketones for its source of fuel. When you eat a no carb diet with high fat, more ketones are being produced. These ketones act as fuel for your brain and improve its functioning. You will see the better focus and mental clarity with time. A carb-loaded diet does the opposite and affects your productivity. Sugars in the diet also have a very negative effect on your gut. The bacteria profile or microbiome content in your gut takes an unhealthy form. When you cut out on these unhealthy sugars, it helps to shift back to the healthy bacteria profile again and the harmful bacteria are eliminated.

The process of burning fats in the body is a continuous process when you are on a high-fat diet. Usually people assume that fats are burned when fats are cut off from the diet; however, the opposite is true. When you are done eating your carnivore diet meal, the body will switch to burning the fat that is stored in the cells already. On a carb diet you have to keep eating to provide your body with fuel to burn. This is why the high-fat diet will keep you feeling energetic all through the day. A high sugar diet is associated with metabolic syndrome. This in turn is linked to heart diseases and diabetes type 2. You will notice excessive weight gain, obesity, high blood pressure, high levels of blood sugar and high triglycerides; the level of good cholesterol of HDL is reduced. Hypertension caused by a high carb diet can be a risk factor for many diseases that primarily affect the heart and kidneys along with other organs. When you eliminate sugars and follow the high-fat carnivore diet, these symptoms will reduce to a healthier state. Reducing carbs will reduce the unhealthy level of triglycerides in your body too. Metabolic syndrome can be very harmful to your body and should be managed with the help of a low carb diet.

One of the main concerns about excessive stored fat in the body is the effect it will have on your health. Especially if the fat is stored in the abdominal cavity. Visceral fat tends to get stored in various organs and affects their functioning. In the abdominal cavity in particular, the visceral fat can cause inflammation, metabolic dysfunction and insulin spikes. This is why low carb intake is recommended to get rid of this fat and thus reduce the risk of the associated diseases.

People assume that eating more carbs will keep them feeling energetic all day. But carbs are just a source of quick boosts of energy. They get burned through fast and you are left with an energy drop constantly. The body finds it very easy to burn carbs and so when this is complete, you will end up feeling hungry again. This is the reason why most people experience hunger pangs on the high carb modern diet. This diet also makes you consume a lot of simple sugars such as fructose, which cause a rise in your triglyceride level. These triglycerides are fat molecules that then increase your risk of cardiovascular diseases. This diet also puts you at higher risk of breast cancer and pancreatic cancer. People who don't pay due attention to the carb intake have more chances of suffering from obesity in the long run. This is why it is important to reduce carbs and monitor the intake level.

Pasta, bread and other products that are grain-based, are all empty carbs. The more you eat the more weight you gain. These empty carbs will not provide your body with energy and just increase your daily calorie intake. Pizza might taste delicious but it is another form of empty calories and is a fast route to gaining more weight. A diet that is based on high carbohydrate intake can even cause nutrient deficiencies. The high-fat meat diet on the other hand will provide you with many important nutrients such as Vitamin E, Vitamin K and Omega 3 fatty acids.

If you see that your body suffers from inflammation most of the time, it is all due to your poor dietary choices. All the unhealthy food that you eat is the main reason behind the inflammation that its results in. Omega 3 fatty acids are anti-inflammatory and these are barely present in the processed foods that you consume daily. Instead your diet has more of omega 6 and there is an unhealthy imbalance due to this. This particular component is usually attained from the various oils you use to cook with such as sunflower oil or soybean oil. These have an inflammatory property unlike omega 3 and the body tends to mobilize these to compounds that are similar to hormones. Trans fat is a bad kind of fat that is found mostly in processed high carb foods. It is very inflammatory and is commonly found in any fried or fast food that you eat. This is why a high junk food diet will cause more inflammation.

Any food that has a very high glycemic index will lead to inflammation at a point. The carbs and refined sugars in your processed foods will increase inflammation. For better health, it is important to eliminate these from your diet. The high glycemic index foods cause an increase in glucose and insulin level that increases inflammation again. Food intolerances are another factor that leads to inflammation and these are usually due to dairy and certain proteins. They will irritate your gut and lead to inflammation. The main culprit behind all this is high carbohydrate intake. If you understand this, you should be more willing to cut out carbs from your diet instead of demonizing fats. Add more healthy fatty foods and you will see effective improvement in your body.

CHAPTER FIFTEEN -

SIDE EFFECTS AND HOW TO DEAL WITH THEM

Following the Ketogenic or the carnivore diet means that you might suffer from a side effect called the Keto-flu. The carnivore diet will definitely be beneficial for your health but the body needs time to get accustomed to the change. You might have to deal with a few side effects such as the Keto flu. In this section, we will explain all about what it is and how you can deal with it.

The Keto flu is actually a common side effect experienced in the initial phase of following the carnivore diet. It is also known as the induction flu and you might experience it within the first week of the transition. The symptoms include nausea, lethargy, headache and lack of concentration. You might find yourself feeling tired all throughout the day; however, thankfully, all this is temporary and can also be prevented. In order to prevent extreme symptoms, you should ensure proper hydration. Drinking adequate water is a very important part of the diet and more so in the adaptation period. Dehydration will cause these symptoms to escalate. Adding a little bit of salt will also help; however, you might also experience some painful leg cramps. These can be a cause of real discomfort since they occur at any time in the day and even while you are sleeping. Drinking a lot of water will cause you to urinate frequently and this causes loss of minerals from your body. This is why leg cramps might occur. But this problem will subside as long as you keep drinking water with a pinch of salt. If it is too much, you should also consider having magnesium supplements but they are not usually required.

Dehydration, mineral loss from frequent urination and eating more dairy products in the diet may also cause constipation. In fact, constipation is also commonly experienced during the first stage. Constipation can be very unhealthy for the body and if it does not pass soon, consult the doctor. Make sure to provide adequate food and liquids to the body to help in the regulation of bowel movements.

The increased production of ketones due to ketosis will also cause acetone breath. Bad breath is one of the more noticeable symptoms that you will have to deal with so try to keep some mints on you. Also ensure that you practice good oral hygiene so that it does not become a serious problem. Some people have also noticed that they experience heart palpitations and shakiness. Diarrhea can also be part of the experience. It is common to see that your sugar cravings reduce but so does your physical performance at the beginning of the diet. To deal with these symptoms, you should consider adding mineral supplements to your diet. These should have sodium, potassium or magnesium. Doctors or dieticians can be consulted to help the transition process easier for you. They will guide you to take the necessary steps to prevent such symptoms. Just remember that all these side effects are temporary, they pass after a while so you just have to endure it for a few days. In the end it gets better and the diet will in fact help you become more energetic and healthier.

The metabolic shift that takes place when you switch from the usual diet to the carnivore diet is what causes the Keto flu. You might experience symptoms like nausea, cramps, night sweats, chills, dry mouth, headaches, dizziness, insomnia and digestive issues. Your level of energy will be low and you might experience brain fog too.

The carnivore diet will help to induce ketosis in the body to help you lose weight. When this happens, the body will start burning fats for energy instead of glucose. While this transition is happening, there will be three significant changes in your body. The fluids in your body will therefore be rebalanced. The insulin level in your body decreases since carbohydrates are eliminated from the diet. Due to this decline in insulin, the kidney will separate sodium from water in your body. The first initial weight loss at the beginning of the diet is just water weight being lost due to this. Then your body will begin emptying its storage of glycogen and after this, fats are burned to gain energy.

Secondly, the body switches to burning fats for energy instead of sugars. Right now your body is used to burning sugars for glucose to get energy. When you start the carnivore diet, it will start burning fats from your food as well as the stored fat in your body and use this as the main source of energy. Each person may react differently to this switch in the energy source. If your body can endure the change well, you will not experience symptoms of Keto flu or at least not too many; however, if this change is harder for your body to deal with, you will experience the distress caused by Keto flu. If you are someone who usually consumes a lot of carbohydrates in your diet, your body is used to using them for energy. This is why it will take the body longer to adapt than some others who may not be as carb dependent as you. In fact, cutting off carbs from your diet might even feel similar to the process of trying to cut off the addiction to caffeine or nicotine.

Thirdly, there is a hormonal rebalance. The level of cortisol and thyroid hormone in your body will undergo some changes in this phase. The thyroid hormone or T3 level in the body will decrease at this point since it is affected by the carbohydrate consumption of a person. These hormones will affect changes in body temperature, heart rate and your metabolism too.

Dealing with the symptoms

It is important to take certain steps to deal with these symptoms. These steps will either help you completely prevent some symptoms or at least decrease the effect they have on your body.

Hydration

One of the most important steps you need to take is to drink adequate water. It is also the easiest to follow so don't overlook this tip to stay hydrated. While you follow the carnivore diet, make sure you drink a minimum of 8 glasses every single day. Water should be something you take in as often as possible. As you already know, processed juices or sodas are not allowed so water is your only bet. Black coffee and tea are permitted but only to a limit. The diet will have a diuretic effect on your body and this will cause a lot of electrolyte loss. In order to replenish this, you need to hydrate constantly. Since the insulin levels also decrease during this diet, the body will excrete even more salts. The lost salt has to be replenished to a healthy level. Just like sugar cravings, sometimes you might feel like you crave something salty. It is your body's way of telling you to replenish the lost salt.

Drinking a lot of water will benefit you in many ways. It will help flush out toxins from your body and your skin will also become much clearer. A high sugar and carb diet have a negative impact on skin and often causes acne. Adequate hydration on the carnivore diet will help to counteract on this. If you don't already have the habit of drinking enough water, set a reminder to help you out initially. Try to drink a glass of water every hour or so. If you want, add some electrolytes to this. Some people also like adding natural flavoring like lemon, cucumber or mint leaves to make them drink more water. These drinks are usually called detox water since the added ingredients contribute anti-oxidants to the water. Adding some flavor is an easy way to trick yourself to stay hydrated. Also drink a glass of water about 30 minutes before every meal you eat. You should also make it as convenient as possible for yourself to drink water. If you move around a lot, just carry a water sipper or bottle with you. It has to be handy so that you don't forget to drink water. Remember to stay away from any sweetened beverages even if they are labeled health drinks. If you drink coffee outside, opt for an Americano and not a Frappuccino. Try and set a goal for drinking water regularly. There are various ways to keep track of your water intake and to keep you motivated. You can keep a diary or just download some apps that have been designed for this very purpose.

Positivity

Positivity will play a big role while you are following the diet and in your life in general. Don't expect instant results and don't let yourself get demotivated. Within a couple of weeks, the body gets adapted and starts showing positive effects of the diet. You should also remember that it is not always the number on the weighing scale that makes a difference. You might be burning fat but gaining muscle so that number might not alter much; however, you can try and keep track of your body measurements that are more likely to change. The fat around your abdominal regions, thighs, etc. will reduce and thus it will change your body size. Use these changes as motivation and be patient to see more impact. You will be pleasantly surprised if you persist in following the diet for long enough. Pictures are also a great way to stay motivated and to track the changed. You can compare the pictures at every stage of the diet and see for yourself how your body has changed for the better.

Stress Management

Dealing with stress is essential. It can be a real hindrance for physical and psychological health. Stress will even hinder the process of inducing ketosis in your body and affect how much fat you can burn. When stress levels rise in the body, there is a natural tendency to crave comfort foods that usually come in the form of sugar or carb-laden foods. This will cause you to break off from the diet and indulge in unhealthy food that will increase your weight again. In order to avoid all this, you have to learn stress management. There are various methods that will help you in doing this, such as meditation or just some hobby. Lower stress levels will ensure better health.

Adequate sleep

Most people of this generation have very unhealthy sleeping habits. They tend to stay awake past midnight and most of the time; it is just while using their smartphones. They then end up oversleeping in the morning or just not getting adequate sleep. Getting a sufficient amount of sleep is essential for being healthy. It also affects your mental health and prevents negative emotions. You should make it a habit of sleeping at a healthy early hour and waking up likewise. You might have a heavy workload but place your health foremost and make some necessary adjustments. Try to be in bed at 10 pm or 11 pm at the most. Getting 7-8 hours of sleep should be a priority. Make sure you can rest undisturbed and at the same hours every night. This will help to restore balance in your circadian rhythm. Use alarms if you cannot do it yourself. Don't waste good hours in the morning in bed and force yourself to get up for a few days. In some time, you will see that it will become a force of habit and you won't even require an alarm. If you find it hard to fall asleep as soon as you are in bed, take time to unwind. Don't play around with your phone. Read a book or listen to some soothing music. Exercising in the evening or going for a walk after dinner will also tire you out and make you sleep better. Regular physical activity has helped a lot of people deal with symptoms of insomnia and regulate sleep; however, it should not be a hectic workout session right before bed since this will release endorphins and adrenaline that will keep you awake. The quality of sleep is very important and even more than the hours you sleep.

Pay attention to the sleep schedule we recommended. Set aside a regular 8 hours at the same time every day. Be consistent in this and you will find it easy in time. Your body will take time to get conditioned to the change in sleep timings. If you find yourself lying awake for an hour while trying to sleep, just get out of bed and do something that helps to soothe you. Then try again and it will get better. Your food and drinks will also affect your sleep quality. Dinner should be eaten a few hours before sleeping and not right before bed; however, don't go to bed feeling hungry either. Eat a little healthy snack if you feel hungry even after dinner but the carnivore diet will usually prevent this and help you feel full. Eating a very heavy meal before bed will also be a cause for discomfort. Also avoid drinking coffee or alcohol before bed. Even nicotine should be consumed with caution if at all since all of these affect your sleep cycle in a negative manner. You should also try drinking more water in the earlier part of the day and not later. Drinking excess water before sleep will disrupt sleep due to frequent urination. The room you sleep in should be conducive to the purpose. Keep it dark and quiet so that it helps you sleep better. Also try to block out any noises and play a soothing instrumental tape to calm you down for a while. If the room is too hot, it will affect your ability to sleep so keep the area cool. Avoid any harsh lighting and also keep the room clean. Avoid sleeping during the day unless you are a child or over 60. You don't really need it but if you do, limit the nap to 30 minutes at most. Napping too much in the day will affect your ability to sleep at night. A bedtime routine will also help you sleep better during the night. Take some time to take care of yourself. A bath, a novel or music will also help to develop a familiar routine to draw you to sleep. Avoid spending hours in bed thinking about stressful things and worrying about your weight, health, or future.

Regular exercise

The carnivore diet by itself will help you in losing a lot of weight and getting fit; however, exercise is always an important part of a healthy lifestyle. Regular exercise will benefit you in more ways than one. You don't have to stress about going to the gym and lifting weight; however, a run in the park or even a brisk walk for 30-40 minutes will benefit you. You can find different ways to stay active every day. Try swimming if you enjoy it and you will see how much faster it helps you burn calories too. You can also go play your favorite sport for a while with your friends like basketball or football or whatever catches your fancy. The main point is to get your body moving and heart rate pumping. Don't make excuses about having a busy schedule, there is always enough time to do these things. Following a properly balanced schedule will help you do everything in its own time. Squeezing in a little time for exercise for your own benefit should not be hard to do. It will strengthen your immune system, release endorphins, help you too lose weight and stay healthy in the long run.

CHAPTER SIXTEEN -

CARNIVORE DIET BREAKFAST RECIPES

Simple Boiled Eggs

Serves: 2

Ingredients:

- 4 eggs
- Water, as required
- Salt to taste (optional)
- Pepper to taste (optional)

Method:

1. Half fill a saucepan with water and place over high heat. When water begins to boil, lower the heat to low heat. Carefully lower the eggs into the pan. Cook until the desired doneness depending on the size of the eggs.
2. **For soft-boiled eggs:** Let the eggs cook for 4-5 minutes.
3. **For medium boiled eggs:** Let the eggs cook for 7-8 minutes.
4. **For hard- boiled eggs:** Cook for 8-10 minutes.
5. Drain and place in a bowl of chilled water.
6. Peel after 4-5 minutes.
7. Season with salt and pepper if desired and serve.

Fried Eggs

Serves: 2

Ingredients:

- 4 eggs
- Salt to taste
- Pepper to taste
- 4 teaspoons butter

Method:

1. Place a nonstick pan over medium heat. Add 1-teaspoon butter and melt. Crack an egg into the pan.
2. **For sunny side up:** Cook until the whites are set and the yolk is runny. Remove with a spatula on to a plate.
3. **For over-easy:** When the whites are set, flip side once. Cook for about 30 seconds and remove on to a plate.
4. **For over- medium:** When the whites are set, flip side once. Cook for about 1 – 1-½ minutes.
5. **For over-hard:** When the whites are set, flip side once. Cook for 2-3 minutes or until the yolk is cooked well, as in a hard- boiled egg.
6. **For steam-fried eggs:** Cook the eggs, sunny side up (step 2) but cover the pan with a lid when the whites are lightly set.
7. Cook the remaining eggs following step 1 and 2 /3/4/5/6
8. Season with salt and pepper and serve.

Soft and Creamy Scrambled Eggs
Serves: 1

Ingredients:

- 2 large free-range eggs
- 1 teaspoon butter
- Salt to taste
- Freshly cracked pepper to taste (optional)

Method:

1. Crack eggs into a bowl. Add and salt and whisk lightly until well combined.
2. Place a nonstick pan over medium heat. Add butter and let it melt. Add the egg mixture. Do not stir for 20 seconds.
3. Using a silicone spatula, stir lightly in small circles for the initial 30 seconds, until slightly curdled.
4. Stir in bigger circles for the next 15 to 20 seconds the egg is curdy in texture. The eggs should be soft and yet set and runny at a few places.
5. Turn off the heat. Let it cook in the heat for 8-10 seconds.
6. Stir lightly. Season with pepper and more salt if desired and serve immediately.

Perfect Scrambled Eggs

Serves: 2

Ingredients:

- 4 large free-range eggs
- 4 tablespoons butter
- ¾ cup single cream or full cream milk
- Salt to taste
- Pepper to taste (optional)

Method:

1. Whisk together eggs in a bowl. Add cream or milk, pepper and salt and whisk until well combined.
2. Place a nonstick pan over medium heat. Add butter. When butter melts, add the egg mixture. Do not stir for 20 seconds.
3. Stir lightly using a wooden spoon. Lift and fold the egg over from the bottom of the pan.
4. Do not stir for another 10 seconds. Lift and fold the egg over from the bottom of the pan.
5. Repeat the previous step until the eggs are cooked soft but also runny at different spots. Turn off the heat.
6. Stir lightly one last time and serve immediately.

Individual Baked Eggs

Serves: 2

Ingredients:

- 2 slices bacon
- 2 eggs
- ½ slice cheddar cheese, cut into 2 halves (in other words two pieces of ¼ slice cheese)
- 2 teaspoons melted butter

Method:

1. Place a deep skillet over medium-high heat. Add cook until brown but yet soft and workable.
2. Remove bacon and place on a plate lined with paper towels.
3. Take 2 muffin cups. Line the inside of each muffin cup with a slice of bacon.
4. Drizzle a teaspoon of butter in each cup.
5. Crack an egg into each cup.
6. Bake in a preheated oven at 350° F for 10-15 minutes depending on how you like it cooked.
7. Place a piece of cheese on top. Bake for some more time until cheese melts.
8. Serve hot.

Scotch Eggs

Serves: 3

Ingredients:

- 3 medium eggs
- ¼ teaspoon salt or to taste
- ½ pound ground or minced pork or beef or lamb or chicken, preferably lean meat
- Pepper to taste (optional)

Method:

1. Half fill a saucepan with water and place over high heat. When water begins to boil, lower the heat to low heat. Carefully lower the eggs into the pan.
2. Let the eggs cook for 4 minutes.
3. Drain and place in a bowl of chilled water.
4. Peel after 4-5 minutes. Dry the eggs by patting with kitchen towels.
5. Add meat (it is better to use lean meat, as the meat may fall apart while baking), salt and pepper into a bowl and mix well. Divide the mixture into 3 equal portions.
6. Take one portion of meat, place on your palm and flatten it. Place one egg in the center and bring the edges together to enclose the egg. Place on a baking sheet, greased with butter.
7. Repeat with the remaining meat and eggs.
8. Bake in a preheated oven at 350° F for 30 minutes depending on how you like it cooked.

Eggs Lorraine

Serves: 1

Ingredients:

- 2 slices Canadian bacon
- 2 eggs
- Salt to taste
- 1 slice Swiss cheese
- 1 tablespoon sour cream
- Pepper to taste

Method:

1. Take a shallow, oval shaped baking dish (of about 1 ½ cups capacity) cups. Line the inside dish with a bacon. Place a cheese slice in the dish.
2. Crack the eggs into the dish.
3. Add sour cream, salt and pepper into a bowl and mix well. Pour into the baking dish.
4. Bake in a preheated oven at 350° F for 10-15 minutes, until the eggs are cooked.
5. Serve hot.

Chicken and Bacon Sausage

Serves: 24

Ingredients:

- 4 large chicken breasts or 2 pounds ground chicken
- 2 eggs, beaten
- 4 slices bacon, cooked, crumbled
- Salt to taste
- Pepper to taste

Method:

1. Add all the ingredients into the food processor bowl. Process until well combined.
2. Divide the mixture into 24 equal portions and shape into patties of about ½ inch thickness.
3. Place the patties on a baking sheet lined with foil.
4. Bake in a preheated oven at 425° F for 20-25 minutes depending on how you like it cooked.
5. Remove from the oven and cool completely. It can be frozen or refrigerated until use.

CHAPTER SEVENTEEN -

CARNIVORE DIET SNACK RECIPES

Devilled Eggs

Serves: 2

Ingredients:

- 4 eggs
- Water, as required
- Salt or Himalayan pink salt to taste
- Pepper to taste (optional)
- 2 tablespoons crumbled cheese

Method:

1. Half fill a saucepan with water and place over high heat. When water begins to boil, lower the heat to low heat. Carefully lower the eggs into the pan. Cook for 8-10 minutes.
2. Drain and place in a bowl of chilled water.
3. Peel after 4-5 minutes.
4. Halve the eggs lengthwise. Carefully scoop the yolks from the eggs and place in a bowl.
5. Add salt, pepper and cheese and mash well. Fill the mixture into the cavity of the yolks with a spoon or transfer the mixture into a piping bag and pipe it into the cavities.
6. Serve as it is or chill and serve later.

Meatballs

Serves: 4-5

Ingredients:

- 2 1/4 pounds ground beef
- 1 teaspoon salt
- 6 tablespoons, grated parmesan cheese
- 1 teaspoon pepper

Method:

1. Add all the ingredients into a bowl and mix until well combined.
2. Make small balls of the mixture and place on a lined baking sheet.
3. Bake in a preheated oven at 350 ° F for about 20-30 minutes depending on the size of the meatballs. Turn the balls around a couple of times while baking.
4. Alternately, place the meatballs in a skillet and cover with a lid. Cook until done. Turn the balls around a couple of times.

Cheese and Meat Roll Ups

Serves: 4

Ingredients:

- 4 slices cooked turkey
- 4 slices cheese

Method:

1. Place turkey slices on a serving platter. Place a slice of cheese on each. Roll and place with the seam sides facing down. Fasten with toothpick if desired and serve.

Roasted Bone Marrow

Serves: 4

Ingredients:

- 8 bone marrow halves
- Freshly ground pepper to taste
- Sea salt flakes

Method:

1. Take a rimmed baking sheet and place the bone marrow halves on it, with the marrow facing up.
2. Bake in a preheated oven at 350 ° F for about 20 to 25 minutes until crisp and golden brown. Most of the fat will be released.
3. Sprinkle salt and pepper to taste and serve.

Pepperoni Meatballs

Serves: 8

Ingredients:

- 2 pounds ground beef or chicken
- 1 teaspoon salt or to taste
- 1 teaspoon pepper or to taste
- 2 eggs, whisked
- ½ pound pepperoni slices, ground or minced

Method:

1. Add all the ingredients into a bowl and mix until well combined.
2. Make small balls of the mixture and place on a lined baking sheet.
3. Bake in a preheated oven at 350 ° F for about 20-30 minutes depending on the size of the meatballs. Turn the balls around a couple of times while baking.
4. Alternately, place the meatballs in a skillet and cover with a lid. Cook until done. Turn the balls around a couple of times.

Liver Burgers

Serves: 7-8

Ingredients:

- 1 pound grass fed beef
- ½ teaspoon pepper
- ½ pound ground liver, drain excess blood

Method:

1. Add all the ingredients into a bowl and mix using your hands.
2. Make 7-8 equal portions of the mixture and shape into patties.
3. Grill on a preheated gill on both the sides until the desired doneness is achieved and serve.

CHAPTER EIGHTEEN -

CARNIVORE DIET SOUP AND BROTH RECIPES

Japanese Tonkotsu Ramen Broth

Serves: 8

Ingredients:

- 1 ¼ pounds pork bones, without any meat
- 1 ¼ pounds pig trotters, only leg portion
- Bones of 1 whole chicken
- 5 1/3 ounces pork skin (optional)
- 8 quarts water + extra to blanch

Method:

1. Chop the larger bones into smaller pieces.
2. To blanch the bones: Take a large pot. Place trotters and all the bones in it. Pour enough water to cover the bones.
3. Place the pot over medium heat. Bring to a boil. Boil for 10 minutes. Remove from heat. Remove the bones and keep it aside.
4. Discard the water and rinse the pot well.
5. Clean the bones of any blood clots with a sharp knife.
6. Add the bones back to the pot along with pork skin. Add 8 quarts of water to it. Bring to a boil.

7. Lower heat and let it simmer.
8. Initially scum will start floating. Remove the scum with a large spoon and discard. Trim the excess fat too.
9. Cover and simmer for about 12- 15 hours. The stock would have reduced in quantity and will be thicker.
10. Remove from heat. When it cools down, strain into a large jar with a wire mesh strainer.
11. Refrigerate for 5-6 days. Unused broth can be frozen.
12. To serve: Heat thoroughly. Add salt and pepper to taste and serve.

Iced Bone Broth

Serves:

Ingredients:

- 2 pounds bones, preferably with a little meat on them
- Water, as required
- Himalayan pink salt to taste

Method:

1. Place bones in a pot. Fill the pot with water (at least 5 quarts). Add 1-teaspoon salt.
2. Place the pot over medium heat. Bring to a boil. Boil for 5 minutes. Cover with a lid. Lower the heat and simmer for 4-5 hours.
3. When the broth is ready, remove the meat if any and use.
4. Strain the broth and cool completely. Use as required.
5. For iced broth: Fill glasses with crushed ice. Pour broth into the glasses and serve.
6. Pour leftovers in a jar and refrigerate until use.

Bacon Cheeseburger Soup

Serves: 2

Ingredients:

- ½ pound ground beef
- 2 cups bone broth
- Salt to taste
- Pepper to taste (optional)
- ¼ cup heavy cream
- ¼ cup bacon bits
- ½ cup milk
- 1 cup cheddar cheese, shredded

Method:

1. Place a soup pot over medium heat. Add bacon and cook until brown and crisp.
2. Add beef and cook until brown. Break it simultaneously as it cooks.
3. Stir in the broth, milk, salt and pepper.
4. When it begins to boil, lower the heat and simmer for 8-10 minutes.
5. Turn off the heat. Add cheese and cream and stir until cheese melts completely.
6. Ladle into soup bowls and serve.

Egg Drop Soup

Serves: 2

Ingredients:

- 3 cups chicken bone broth
- 1 egg beaten
- Salt to taste
- Pepper to taste

Method:

1. Boil broth in a saucepan.
2. When the broth begins to boil, lower the heat.
3. Pour the egg, in a thin stream into the broth stirring simultaneously. Stir only in one direction.
4. Turn off the heat. Let it sit for a minute.
5. Ladle into soup bowls. Season with salt and pepper to taste.

Creamy Chicken Soup

Serves: 8

Ingredients:

- 4 tablespoons butter
- 8 ounces cream cheese, cubed
- 4 cup chicken bone broth
- Salt to taste
- Pepper to taste
- 4 cups cooked, shredded chicken breast
- ½ cup heavy cream

Method:

1. Place a saucepan over medium heat. Add butter and butter melt. Add chicken and sauté for a couple of minutes until the chicken is well coated with the butter.
2. Add cream cheese and mix well.
3. When cream cheese melts, add broth and cream and stir.
4. Add salt and pepper and stir.
5. Ladle into soup bowls and serve.

Cheddar Chicken Soup

Serves: 8

Ingredients:

- 1 pound chicken breasts, skinless, boneless, chopped into bite size chunks
- 4 cups milk
- 2 cups shredded cheddar cheese
- 6 cups chicken broth
- Salt to taste
- 1 tablespoon butter

Method:

1. Place a saucepan over medium heat. Add butter and butter melt. Add chicken and sauté for a couple of minutes until the chicken is well coated with the butter.
2. Stir in the broth and milk. Cook until chicken is tender.
3. Turn off the heat.
4. Add cheese and salt and stir until cheese melts.
5. Ladle into soup bowls and serve.

CHAPTER NINETEEN –

CARNIVORE DIET POULTRY RECIPES

Salt and Pepper Turkey

Serves: 5-8

Ingredients:

- 1 whole turkey of about 9-10 pounds, discard giblets
- 3-5 tablespoons butter
- Coarse salt to taste
- Freshly ground pepper to taste

Method:

1. Pour 2 cups water in a large roasting pan. Place a rack in the pan.
2. Start at the neck and loosen the skin on the breast area. Take some of the butter and rub it beneath the skin.
3. Sprinkle salt and pepper, generously all over the turkey and the cavity. Using a thick kitchen string, tie up the legs together. Place turkey on the rack and tuck the wings below.
4. Bake in a preheated oven at 350 ° F for 2-3 hours or until the internal temperature when checked with an instant read thermometer in the thickest part of the meat shows 165 ° F.

5. Baste the turkey with remaining butter after every 25 to 30 minutes. Slightly shake the turkey so that the cooked juice falls into the pan.

6. Remove turkey from the oven and place on your cutting board. Tent with foil and let it sit for 30 minutes.

7. When cool enough to handle, cut into slices. Drizzle some of the cooked liquid from the pan over the turkey and serve.

Turkey in Cream Sauce

Serves: 4

Ingredients:

- 3 tablespoons butter
- ¾ cup heavy cream
- Salt to taste
- Pepper to taste
- ¾ cup chicken stock
- 2 cups cooked, chopped turkey

Method:

1. Place a large pan over medium heat. Add butter and cook until it turns golden in color.
2. Add stock and simmer for 5-6 minutes.
3. Add cream, turkey, salt and pepper. Simmer for a few minutes.
4. Serve hot.

Turkey with Cheddar Cheese Sauce

Serves: 2

Ingredients:

- 4 slices (1 ounce each) cooked turkey breast
- 2 tablespoons butter + extra to grease
- ½ cup milk or half and half
- Pepper to taste
- Salt to taste
- ½ cup shredded cheddar cheese

Method:

1. Take a small square baking dish of about 6x6 inches and grease with a little butter.
2. Lay the turkey slices in the dish.
3. Place a saucepan over medium heat. Add butter and melt.
4. Add turkey, salt, pepper and half and half and simmer for a couple of minutes.
5. Add cheese and cook until it melts and well blended with the other ingredients.
6. Turn off the heat.
7. Pour over the turkey.
8. Bake in a preheated oven at 350 ° F for about 20 minutes or until the sauce is bubbling.

Duck Leg Confit

Serves: 2

Ingredients:

- 2 duck legs with thigh, trimmed of excess fat and retain it
- 3-5 tablespoons butter
- Table salt to taste
- ½ tablespoon kosher salt
- Freshly ground pepper to taste
- 2 cups duck fat (that was retained)
- ¾ teaspoon whole peppercorns

Method:

1. Place the duck legs on a large plate, with the skin side facing down. Season with kosher salt and pepper.
2. Pour the duck fat in a baking dish.
3. Stack the duck legs in the baking dish and place in the refrigerator for 10 to 12 hours.
4. Remove the duck and rinse in cold water. Lightly wipe off the salt and pepper.
5. Dry with paper towels.
6. Remove the duck fat and place in an enameled cast iron pot.
7. Scatter peppercorns on the fat. Sprinkle salt over it.
8. Place the duck, with the skin side facing down in the pot. Place some duck fat on top of the duck. Cover and place in a preheated oven.
9. Bake at 350 ° F for about 2-3 hours or until the meat falls away from the bone.

10. Strain the fat from the dish into a bowl. Retain the fat to store meat or use in some other recipe.

11. If you want serve right away, transfer the duck legs into a pan, with the skin side facing down. Place the pan over medium high heat and sear until the skin is crisp and brown.

12. If you want to eat after a few days, remove the meat from the bones and keep it in a stoneware container. Pour some of the retained fat over the meat. (Fat should cover by at least ¼ inch over the meat). Place the container in the refrigerator until use. It can last for a month.

Crispy Chicken Thighs

Serves: 4-8

Ingredients:

- 6 chicken thighs, with skin
- 2 tablespoons butter or lard, melted
- Freshly ground pepper to taste
- Kosher salt to taste

Method:

1. Dry the chicken by patting with paper towels. Season with salt and pepper.
2. Toss well.
3. Place the chicken pieces on a baking sheet with the skin side facing up, in a single layer. Drizzle butter over it
4. Roast in a preheated oven at 400 ° F for 20 – 30 minutes or until cooked through. The internal temperature in the thickest part of the meat should show 165 ° F.
5. If you want the skin to be crisp, broil for a couple of minutes.

BBQ Chicken Livers and Hearts

Serves: 4-6

Ingredients:

- 2 pounds chicken livers, thawed to room temperature
- 2 pounds chicken hearts, thawed to room temperature
- Pepper to taste
- Salt to taste
- A few bamboo skewers, soaked in water for an hour

Method:

1. Clear the excess fat from the hearts and livers and clean them too.
2. Place them flat, in a flexible grilling basket.
3. Sprinkle salt and pepper over the meat.
4. Grill on a charcoal grill until the way you like it cooked.

Chicken with Cheesy Sauce

Serves: 3

Ingredients:

- 6 chicken thighs
- ½ teaspoon pepper
- ½ teaspoon salt
- 1 cup chicken bone broth
- 4 ounces cream cheese
- ½ cup heavy cream
- 10 tablespoons butter, divided
- 1 cup mozzarella cheese, shredded

Method:

1. Place a large skillet over medium heat. Add 2 tablespoons butter and allow it to melt.
2. Sprinkle salt and pepper over the chicken. Sprinkle beneath the skin also.
3. Place chicken in the skillet with the skin side facing down.
4. Cover and cook for 6 minutes or until the skin side is brown. Remove chicken with a slotted spoon and set aside on a plate.
5. Pour broth into the skillet. Scrape the bottom of the pan to remove any browned bits that may be stuck.
6. Add chicken back into the pan. Cover and cook until chicken is cooked through.
7. Meanwhile, make the sauce as follows: Add cream cheese, cream and remaining butter into a saucepan. Place saucepan over low heat.

8. Stir constantly until the mixture is well incorporated. Turn off the heat.
9. Whisk in the mozzarella cheese. Stir constantly until cheese melts.
10. Place chicken in bowls. Pour cheesy sauce over it and serve.

Salt and Pepper Roast Chicken

Serves: 4-8

Ingredients:

- 2-3 pounds chicken, cut into parts (bone-in and skin on if using chicken breasts)
- Freshly ground pepper to taste
- Kosher salt to taste

Method:

1. Dry the chicken by patting with paper towels. You can also use whole chicken. Place in a bowl.
2. Sprinkle salt and pepper over the chicken. Chill for 1-8 hours.
3. Place the chicken pieces in a roasting pan, with the skin side facing up, in a single layer.
4. Roast in a preheated oven at 400 ° F for about 30 minutes (or 50-60 minutes if using whole chicken) or until cooked through. The internal temperature in the thickest part of the meat should show 165 ° F.
5. If you want the skin to be crisp, broil for a couple of minutes.
6. If using whole chicken, remove from the oven and cool for a while. Slice and serve.

Parmesan Crusted Chicken Thighs with Bacon Cream Sauce

Serves: 2

Ingredients:

For Parmesan crusted chicken:

- 4 chicken thighs
- ½ cup freshly grated parmesan cheese
- ¼ teaspoon salt
- 2 -3 tablespoons butter, melted
- ¼ teaspoon pepper (optional)

For bacon cream sauce:

- 3 slices bacon
- ½ tablespoon sour cream
- ¼ cup heavy whipping cream
- ½ tablespoon shredded parmesan cheese

Method:

1. Add melted butter in a shallow bowl.
2. Place salt, pepper and Parmesan cheese on a plate. Mix well.
3. Dip a chicken thigh in butter. Shake to drop off excess butter. Dredge in the Parmesan and place in a greased baking dish with the skin side facing up.
4. Repeat with the remaining chicken thighs.
5. Bake in a preheated oven at 400 ° F for about 35- 50 minutes depending on the size of the thighs.

6. For bacon cream sauce: Place a skillet over medium heat.
7. Add bacon and cook until crisp. Remove with a slotted spoon (retain the bacon fat in the pan) and set aside on a plate. When cool enough to handle, crumble the bacon.
8. Add cream into the skillet and whisk until well blended.
9. Continue whisking until tiny bubbles appear on the edges of the pan.
10. Whisk in the sour cream.
11. Divide the chicken into 2 plates. Divide the sauce among the plates and serve.

Simple, Pan-fried Chicken Breasts

Serves: 4-5

Ingredients:

- 8 chicken breast halves
- 2 tablespoons butter or lard
- Freshly ground pepper to taste
- Kosher salt to taste
- ¼ cup grated parmesan cheese (optional)

Method:

1. Place a stainless steel or cast – iron skillet over medium heat. Add butter or lard and let the pan heat.
2. Using a meat mallet, pound the chicken breast until the chicken is uniformly thick.
3. Season with salt and pepper if using. Let it rest for 15-20 minutes.
4. Place an ovenproof skillet over high heat. Place chicken in the skillet.
5. Cook for 2-3 minutes without stirring or covering. Cook until golden brown and the fat is released. Flip sides cook for 2-3 minutes.
6. Remove from the heat and garnish with Parmesan cheese.
7. Broil for 2-3 minutes and serve.

Chicken with Creamy Bacon Sauce

Serves: 10

Ingredients:

- 10 chicken thighs
- ½ teaspoon pepper
- ½ teaspoon salt
- 1 cup chicken bone broth
- 1 cup double heavy cream
- 4 tablespoons butter, softened
- 16 slices bacon

Method:

1. Place a pan over medium heat. Add bacon and cook until brown. Drain the fat remaining in the pan. When cool enough to handle, chop into small pieces. Set aside.
2. Place a large skillet over medium heat. Add butter and melt.
3. Sprinkle salt and pepper over the chicken. Sprinkle beneath the skin as well.
4. Place chicken in the skillet with the skin side facing down.
5. Cover and cook for 6 minutes or until the skin side is brown. Remove chicken with a slotted spoon and set aside on a plate.
6. Pour broth into the skillet. Scrape the bottom of the pan to remove any browned bits that may be stuck.
7. Add chicken back into the pan. Add half the bacon. Cover and cook until chicken is cooked through. Remove chicken with a slotted spoon and set aside.

8. Add cream and remaining butter into the same skillet.
9. Stir constantly until the mixture is well incorporated.
10. Add chicken back into the skillet and mix well. Simmer for a couple of minutes. Turn off the heat.
11. Place chicken in bowls. Sprinkle remaining bacon on top and serve.

Easy Chicken Salad

Serves: 4-5

Ingredients:

- 1 cup sour cream
- 4-5 chicken breast halves
- Salt to taste
- Pepper to taste
- 1 cup feta cheese, crumbled
- 4 slices bacon
- 4 hard-boiled eggs, peeled, quartered

Method:

1. Place the chicken in a stockpot. Cover with cold water. Sprinkle salt.
2. Place the stockpot over medium heat. Cook until chicken is tender. Remove the chicken with a pair of tongs and place on your cutting board. Shred or chop into pieces.
3. Place a pan over medium heat. Add bacon and cook until brown.
4. Remove with a slotted spoon and place on a plate lined with paper towels. When cool enough to handle, chop into pieces.
5. Add chicken, bacon, and rest of the ingredients into a bowl and fold gently.
6. Chill and serve.

CHAPTER TWENTY -

CARNIVORE DIET SEAFOOD RECIPES

Baked Fish Fillets

Serves: 3

Ingredients:

- 2-3 tablespoons melted butter + extra to grease
- 1-pound mackerel fillets
- Pepper to taste
- ½ teaspoon salt

Method:

1. Grease a baking dish with a little butter. Lay the fillets in the dish. Sprinkle salt and pepper over it.
2. Drizzle melted butter over the fillets.
3. Bake in a preheated oven at 350 ° F for about 20 to 25 minutes or until the fish flakes easily when pierced with a fork.
4. Serve hot.

Perfect Grilled Fish Fillets

Serves: 2-3

Ingredients:

- 2 large white fish fillets
- ½ teaspoon freshly ground pepper
- ¾ teaspoon kosher salt + extra to garnish
- 4 tablespoons melted butter

Method:

1. Clean and rinse the fillets and place over layers of paper towels. Also pat the fillets dry with paper towels.
2. Sprinkle half the salt and half the pepper on the fillets. Pour half the butter over the fish. Brush the butter over the fillets.
3. Turn the sides of the fillet and sprinkle remaining salt and pepper over it. Pour remaining butter and brush over the fillets.
4. Preheat a grill to high heat for 5-10 minutes. Clean the grill grate and lower the heat to low heat.
5. Place fillets on the grill and cover with the lid. Grill for 7-10 minutes or until it flakes easily when pierced with a fork.
6. Sprinkle some more salt on top and serve.

Grilled Split Lobster

Serves: 4-6

Ingredients:

- 4 tablespoons melted butter + extra to serve and grease
- Kosher salt to taste
- Freshly ground pepper to taste
- 4 live lobsters (1 ½ pounds each)

Method:

1. Preheat a grill to high heat for 5-10 minutes. Clean the grill grate and lower the heat to low heat.
2. Place lobsters in the freezer for 15 minutes.
3. Hold the tail. Split the lobsters in half lengthwise. Start from the point where tail joins the body and up to the head. Flip sides and halve it lengthwise via the tail.
4. Rub melted butter on the cut part, immediately after cutting. Sprinkle salt and pepper over it.
5. Place on the grill and press the claws on the grill until cooked. Grill for 6-8 minutes.
6. Flip side and cook until it is cooked through and lightly charred.
7. Serve right out of the grill with melted butter on top.

Grilled Fillet with Blue Cheese Butter

Serves: 2

Ingredients:

- 4 tablespoon butter, slightly softened
- Salt to taste
- Freshly cracked pepper to taste
- Melted butter, to brush
- 2-3 tablespoons crumbled Cabrales blue cheese
- 2 fillet mignons (1 ½ inches thick)

Method:

1. Add butter, salt, pepper and cheese into a bowl and stir. Cover and chill for 30 minutes.
2. Brush steaks with melted butter. Sprinkle salt and pepper over the steak.
3. Place on a preheated grill (heated to high heat) and grill on both the sides until medium – rare and charred.
4. Remove the steaks and place on plate.
5. Spread the blue cheese butter over it.
6. Serve after 5 minutes.

CHAPTER TWENTY-ONE -

CARNIVORE DIET MEAT (BEEF, LAMB, PORK ETC.) RECIPES

Baked / Broiled Steak

Serves: 1

Ingredients:

- 1 strip loin steaks (10-12 ounces), 1 ½ inches thick, at room temperature
- ¼ teaspoon kosher salt
- 1 tablespoon butter or lard, melted
- Freshly ground pepper to taste (optional)

Method:

1. Dry the steak by patting with paper towels.
2. **For roasting in an oven:** Brush ½ tablespoon butter over the steak and rub it well into it. Sprinkle salt and pepper if using.
3. Place a skillet over medium heat. When the pan heats, place steak in the skillet and cook for a minute. Flip sides and cook for a minute.
4. Place a rack on a rimmed baking sheet.
5. Place steak on the rack. Place baking sheet in the oven.

6. Roast in a preheated oven at 375 ° F:
7. For rare: Roast for 10 minutes and internal temperature should be 120 ° F.
8. For medium: Roast for 14 minutes and internal temperature should be 145 ° F.
9. For well cooked: Roast for 18 minutes and internal temperature should be 155 ° F.
10. **For broiling in an oven:** After step 2, place steak in a broiling pan. You can also keep on a rack.
11. Place the broiling pan 6 inches away from the heating element.
12. For rare: Broil for 2 minutes. Flip once and broil for 2 minutes.
13. For medium: Broil for 4 minutes. Flip once and broil for minutes.
14. For well cooked: Broil for 6 minutes. Flip once and broil for 6 minutes.
15. Serve hot.

Liver Bacon Meatballs

Serves: 6

Ingredients:

- 1 pound grass-fed and finished beef liver, thawed
- 3 pounds grass-fed and finished ground beef
- 16 ounces organic, uncured bacon, chopped into small pieces
- ½ cup cream from top of raw milk
- 2 eggs
- Sea salt to taste
- Freshly ground pepper to taste

Method:

1. Place a large pan over medium heat. Add bacon and cook until brown but not too crisp.
2. Remove bacon with a slotted spoon and place on a plate lined with layers of paper towels.
3. When bacon cools, transfer into the food processor bowl and process until crumbly. Add liver into the food processor bowl. Continue processing until it is liquid in texture.
4. Add eggs, salt, pepper and cream into a bowl and whisk well. Pour into the food processor bowl. Also add beef and pulse until well combined.
5. Make small balls of the mixture.
6. Heat the same pan in which bacon was cooked. Add meatballs and cook until brown all over (2-3 minutes on each side). Cover and cook until the meat inside is

well cooked. Add more butter or lard if required will frying.

7. Serve hot.

Carnivore Burger

Serves: 8

Ingredients:

- 2 pounds ground beef
- 2 pounds ground bison
- 2 pounds ground lamb
- 2 pounds ground pork
- 8 large eggs
- Salt to taste (optional)
- Pepper to taste (optional)

Method:

1. Preheat grill to high heat.
2. Add all the meat and eggs into a large bowl and mix well using your hands.
3. Divide the mixture into 8 equal portions. Shape into patties of about 1 inch thickness. Season with salt and pepper if desired.
4. Place 2-3 burgers on the preheated grill. Grill for 5-7 minutes. Flip sides and cook for 5-7 minutes. The internal temperature of the burger should be around 135 ° F when checked with a meat thermometer. Grill in batches.
5. Remove the burgers from the grill and place on a plate. Tent with foil for 5 minutes.
6. Serve.

Carnivore Meatloaf

Serves: 2-4

Ingredients:

- 2 pounds ground pork (80/20)
- 4 pounds ground beef (80/20)
- Salt to taste

Method:

1. Add beef into a mixing bowl. Add salt and mix with your hands until well combined.
2. Add pork and knead until well combined.
3. Transfer into a rectangular baking dish. Press it well onto the bottom of the dish.
4. Bake in a preheated oven at 350 ° F for about 30-40 minutes or until the cooked juices are released in the center and it looks cooked at the edges. The edges will begin to leave the dish.
5. Remove from the oven.
6. Cool for a while. Cut into slices and serve.

Parmesan Butter Pork Chops

Serves: 2

Ingredients:

- 4 pork chops
- 4-5 tablespoons butter
- 5-6 tablespoons powdered parmesan cheese
- Salt to taste

Method:

1. Place a large skillet over medium heat. Add butter. When butter melts, place the pork chops and cook until light brown on both the sides. Transfer the pork chops into a baking dish.
2. Drizzle butter over the pork chops. Sprinkle salt and Parmesan cheese powder.
3. Cover the dish with foil.
4. Bake in a preheated oven at 275 ° F for about 30 minutes.

50/50/50 Burgers

Serves: 6-8

Ingredients:

- 2 pounds ground beef or any other meat of your choice
- 2 pounds bacon
- 2 pounds bison liver or any other liver of your choice

Method:

1. Add bacon and liver into the food processor bowl and process until liver becomes almost liquid.
2. Transfer into a bowl. Add ground beef and mix well.
3. Divide the mixture into 8-ounce portions and shape into patties.
4. Grill the burgers on a preheated grill or cook in a pan using some lard or butter.
5. You can also bake in a preheated oven at 400 ° F for about 18-20 minutes according to the desired doneness.

Perfect Skillet Steak

Serves: 1-2

Ingredients:

- Steak of 7/8 thickness
- Butter or lard, melted, to brush
- Salt to taste
- Pepper to taste

Method:

1. Place a skillet over medium high heat and allow it to heat.
2. Brush steak with butter and place on the skillet.
3. _For rare:_ Cook for 2-3 minutes. Flip sides once and cook side for 2-3 minutes. Using a pair of tongs (back part), press the steak in the center. If it is soft, turn off the heat.
4. _For medium:_ Cook for 4 minutes. Flip side once and cook the other side for 4 minutes. Using a pair of tongs (back part), press the steak in the center. If it is slightly firmer, turn off the heat.
5. _For well cooked:_ Cook for 5-6 minutes. Flip side once and cook the other side for 5-6 minutes. Using a pair of tongs (back part), press the steak in the center. If it is very firm, turn off the heat.
6. When the steak is cooked as per your liking, remove steak from the pan and place on a plate. Tent with foil and let it rest for 5 minutes.
7. Slice and serve. Season with salt and pepper if desired.

Pan Seared Beef Tongue

Serves: 2

Ingredients:

- 2 whole beef tongues, rinsed
- 2 tablespoons lard or butter
- 3 cups water

Method:

1. Pour water into a saucepan. Add tongues and place saucepan over medium heat.
2. When it begins to boil, lower the heat to low heat. Cover and cook until tender. Alternately, you can cook it in a pressure cooker.
3. Remove tongues and place on your cutting board. When cool enough to handle, cut into slices.
4. Place a pan over medium heat. Add butter and melt. Place tongue slices and sear for 2-3 minutes. Flip sides and cook the other side for 2-3 minutes.
5. Serve hot.

CONCLUSION

As you have come to the end of this book, we would first like to thank you for using this source for learning more about the carnivore diet. We hope you gained enough information to understand the pros and cons of following this meat only diet. We are sure that any meat lovers reading this book will definitely give it a go.

If you want to learn more from people who have already tried the diet, there are various online communities that you can find online. You can also consult your doctor while deciding if the diet is appropriate for you; however, more often than not, this diet is suitable and effective for you especially in terms of weight loss. The first week or so of starting the diet might seem a little tough to get through but you need to persevere through it.

After these initial days pass, the diet becomes very easy to follow and you will get used to it. While following the diet, track your progress and measure it quantitatively as well as qualitatively. Use this book as a guide while trying the carnivore diet and see how it works for you. If you find it useful, you can also go ahead and share or recommend it to family or friends who might benefit from following the carnivore diet too.